Advance Praise for Sp

"A practical book by a practical doc. This is good reading for anyone who has heartburn or takes care of heartburn patients."
— *Joel E. Richter, MD, FACP, MACG, Professor of Medicine and Chairman, Department of Medicine, Temple University School of Medicine*

"Dr. Challa's new book Spurn the Burn will undoubtedly become a bible for all those millions suffering from acid reflux disease"
— *Prof. Dr. Michael Nobel, Chairman, Nobel Family Association, Stockholm, Sweden*

"Dr. Challa's book offers a comprehensive overview of gastroesophageal reflux disease and its treatment, including various herbal remedies."
— *The National Heartburn Alliance*

"Dr. Challa has written an invaluable resource for acid reflux suffers. He guides the reader through the new advances in diagnostics, signs and symptoms, complications, and treatment options with a command of the topic and an understanding of how people really think and live."
— *Elaine Magee, MPH, RD, The Recipe Doctor and author of 25 books, including* Tell Me What to Eat If I Have Acid Reflux *and* Fry Light, Fry Right!

"Anyone who's ever suffered from acid reflux must read this book. Dr. Challa explains in simple detail how you can change and improve the quality of your life. Take control of your health and read this book today."
— *Sally Taylor, author of the award-winning* On My Own

Spurn the Burn

◯ ▯ ✐ ▭ **My Healing Helpers**

Introducing the latest GERD technology — Find the enemy with PillCam

Spurn the Burn

Treat the Heat

Everything you need to know to beat ACID REFLUX DISEASE

from the award-winning author of *Winning the Hepatitis C Battle*

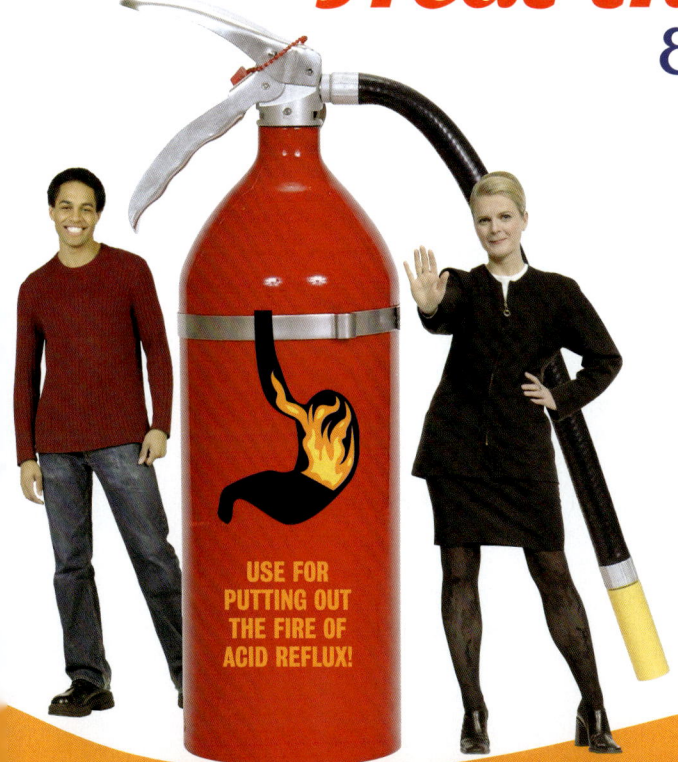

USE FOR PUTTING OUT THE FIRE OF ACID REFLUX

Shekhar Challa, MD

Topeka, KS

Spurn the Burn, Treat the Heat:
Everything You Need to Know to Beat Acid Reflux Disease
by Shekhar Challa, M.D.

Published 2005 by Kansas Medical Publishing
2200 SW 6th Street, Topeka, KS 66606
For ordering information, visit www.spurntheburn.com or call (866) 746-1448.

Copyright © 2005 by Shekhar Challa, M.D. All Rights Reserved. No part of this book may be reproduced or transmitted in any form or by any means, graphic, electronic, or mechanical, including photocopying, recording, taping, or by any information storage or retrieval system – except by a reviewer who may quote brief passages in a review to be printed in a magazine, newspaper, or on the web – without written permission from the publisher.

Cover and interior design by Pneuma Books, LLC
For more info, visit www.pneumabooks.com

10 09 08 07 06 05   6 5 4 3 2 1

Publisher's Cataloging-In-Publication
(Prepared by Quality Books, Inc.)

       Challa, Shekhar.
         Spurn the burn, treat the heat : everything you need to know to beat acid reflux disease / Shekhar Challa. -- 1st ed.
         p. cm.
         Includes index.
         LCCN 2004118111
         ISBN-13: 978-0-9743883-3-5
         ISBN-10: 0-9743883-3-5

        1. Gastroesophageal reflux--Popular works.
       I. Title.

RC815.7.C43 2005   616.3'24
                          QBI05-200058

Disclaimer

All information contained in any Kansas Medical Publishing publications, including all designs, text, graphics, the selection and arrangement thereof, are owned or controlled by Kansas Medical Publishing or its affiliates and protected by worldwide copyright laws. Permission to use, copy, or distribute any such information without compensation is hereby granted for non-commercial personal use only, provided the information is not modified, reused, reposted, or retransmitted, and the copyright and other intellectual property notices appear in all copies. Under no circumstances may the name of Kansas Medical Publishing or Spurn the Burn be used in any advertising or publicity without the express prior written permission of Kansas Medical Publishing. All images used in any Kansas Medical Publishing publication are owned or licensed by Kansas Medical Publishing and are solely for use in its publications. Unauthorized use is prohibited. Kansas Medical Publishing and its affiliates will aggressively enforce its intellectual property rights in their publications and their contents to the fullest extent of the law.

Kansas Medical Publishing and its affiliates do not represent or warrant that the Kansas Medical Publishing's services will be uninterrupted, error-free, or that defects will be corrected. Kansas Medical Publishing and its affiliates do not warrant or represent that information provided in any Kansas Medical Publishing or its affiliates' publications will be correct, accurate, timely, or otherwise reliable. Kansas Medical Publishing and its affiliates make no warranties, express or implied, concerning the data contained in this disk, or the physical materials and processes used in producing or duplicating the disk. Kansas Medical Publishing and its affiliates expressly disclaim all implied warranties, including but not limited to the implied warranties of merchantability and fitness for a particular purpose.

You are hereby advised and, by use of this work, you specifically agree that Kansas Medical Publishing and its affiliates' publications are not intended to treat, diagnose, cure, or prevent any condition or disease. You should carefully read all information and consult your physician or health care practitioner before making any decision regarding your own or others' healthcare. Although we carefully review our content, Kansas Medical Publishing and its affiliates cannot guarantee, nor do we take responsibility for, the medical accuracy of documents we publish, nor can Kansas Medical Publishing or its affiliates assume any liability for the content of information provided in any of its publications, reliance thereon, or actions taken in reliance thereon.

*To my wife, Jaya, who gives up much
of our time together for my many projects and more...*

Thank you for your unwavering support and love.

Publisher's Preface

It is estimated that an astounding 60,000,000 Americans suffer from heartburn on a monthly basis — sixty million! It is an epidemic and Americans need relief. Pharmaceutical companies and their advertisers understand this well… our drugstore shelves and televisions are packed with remedies and miracle cures. Yet heartburn abounds. And, worse, it is one of the most common symptoms of a disease that can have fatal implications — GERD — Gastroesophageal Reflux Disease.

Consumer ignorance can be deadly. Left untreated, GERD can progress to Barrett's esophagus, dysplasia, and even esophageal cancer. There is hope on the horizon, however, as some recent advances in diagnostic options (namely, the Bravo™ pH Monitoring System and the PillCam™ ESO) and pharmacological treatments available to GERD sufferers should dramatically alter the way both doctors and patients approach GERD treatment.

This book educates consumers on these treatments and other practices. Consumers are now equipped to understand common heartburn so that GERD does not progress to the more serious diseases associated with it. For patients suffering with Barrett's esophagus, dysplasia, and esophageal cancer, this book provides valuable insight into prognosis and treatment.

GERD affects between 5 – 7 percent of the world's population in every age group from infants to geriatrics, every socioeconomic class, and every ethnic group. The United States Department of Health and Human Services estimates that about seven million Americans have been diagnosed with GERD, and one can only speculate as to how many more cases go undiagnosed each year due to ignorance or fear about this chronic disease and its diagnosis.

Kansas Medical Publishing undertook this book project to provide the consumer with easy-to-understand and thorough information about GERD. This book, if used properly, can turn the deadly tide for millions of suffering people.

Dr. Shekhar Challa has been at the forefront of gastroenterology and hepatology for more than eighteen years, and his goal is to educate the general public about GERD — its symptoms, diagnosis, and treatment options — so that many more GERD sufferers will no longer suffer in silence but will consult their doctors and get the help they need in fighting this disease.

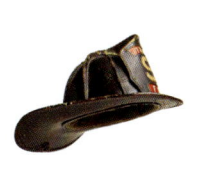

Acknowledgments

This book is written for my patients and the millions of GERD sufferers.

To my daughters, Akhila and Shruti, who make all my work worthwhile. You keep me focused and remind me about the truly important things in life.

To my father, who taught me that hard work, a clear conscience, and persistence lead to success.

To my mother, who has quietly guided me with common sense and love.

To my father-in-law, Dr. Pampati Kishen, who has been a role model since my early childhood. To my brothers — Kishore, Prasanna, Praveen, and Sanjay for giving me a wonderful childhood and being my four best friends for life.

To my nephews, Karthik Challa, Ashwin Pampati, Rudra Pampati, and my niece, Supriya Challa, (all aspiring doctors!) who offered their unstinting help with research for this book.

To my good friend, Dr. Rao Donepudi, for inspiring me to continue writing.

To Morgan and Shelby, for countless meetings, hundreds of emails, and hours of hard work in putting this book together.

To the National Heartburn Alliance, for their willingness to share information and recipes in an effort to challenge the effects GERD has on millions of people.

Contents

Publisher's Preface xi
Acknowledgments xv
Foreword by Dr. Bergein Overholt xxi
Introduction: The Epidemic of a New Millennium xxv

Chapter One: No Respecter of Persons 1
    Faces of GERD 1
    Charles Wurm 1
    Sue Michalski 3
    Jim Cline 5
    Carlene Parks 6

Chapter Two: Burn, Baby, Burn! 9
    The Signs and Symptoms of GERD 9
    Most Common (Typical) GERD Symptoms 10
    Less Common (Atypical) GERD Symptoms 12
    Two Kinds of Reflux Disease 14
    Other Factors that May Aggravate GERD Symptoms 15
    Medications that May Aggravate GERD Symptoms 15

Chapter Three: The Throat Bone's Connected to the Stomach Bone 19
    The Anatomy of GERD 19
    The Normal Digestive Process 20

Other Contributing Factors 22
Hiatal Hernia 24

Chapter Four: What Went Wrong? 27
The Complications of GERD 27
Erosive or Ulcerative Esophagitis 28
Barrett's Esophagus 28
Esophageal Stricture 33
Esophageal Adenocarcinoma (Cancer of the Esophagus) ..34
Uncomfortable but Harmless or Deadly Serious 36

Chapter Five: Open up and Say, "Ah!" 39
The Diagnosis of GERD 39
Esophagogastroduodenoscopy or EGD 41
PillCam ESO 42
The Bravo pH Monitoring System 44
Other Testing Methods 46

Chapter Six: Pills, Knife, or No More Spice 51
Treatment Options for GERD 51
Lifestyle Changes..52
Pharmacological Management or Medical Management ..54
Endoscopic Management 61
Surgical Management 62
Risks and Side Effects of Surgery 64
Treatment Options for the Complications of GERD 65

Chapter Seven: A Spot of Camomile Tea 69
Herbal and Alternative Treatments for GERD 69

Contents

Chapter Eight: Bugs, Mommies, Babies, and Grannies 77
    Helicobacter Pylori and GERD 77
    Pregnancy and GERD 78
    GERD in Infants and Children 79
    GERD and the Elderly..79

Afterword 83
Frequently Asked Questions..........................87
Glossary 95
Recipes Amenable to GERD Sufferers 103
Recommended Websites 125

Index 129
Special Thanks..137
About the Author 141

Foreword

By Dr. Bergein Overholt

When I began practicing medicine over thirty years ago, there were very few options that I could offer patients who complained of severe heartburn or who were diagnosed with GERD, gastroesophageal reflux disease. For some people with significant problems, we offered treatments that were, overall, not very effective.

That certainly is not true today. Over the years, I have seen a tremendous increase in the incidence of GERD, something that I attribute to lifestyle and dietary changes.

Thankfully, the medical field has been able to respond to this problem with effective medications that can control the effect GERD and its associated symptoms have on the patient's quality of life. In particular, the introduction of proton pump inhibitors changed everything about treatment in this field, becoming almost a "magic medicine." It was a relief to be able to offer patients such a successful option to treat heartburn.

While I've been extremely grateful for pharmaceutical advances that give patients relief, I've also been concerned that the availability of effective over-the-counter medicines keeps them from seeking professional medical advice about GERD. I have found that many patients are unaware that GERD can lead to a pre-cancerous condition called Barrett's Esophagus, which in turn can become deadly esophageal cancer.

It is as straightforward as this — without a medical diagnosis, you cannot be sure that you're receiving proper treatment. If acid reflux is identified early enough, there is a good possibility that Barrett's can be prevented. And if Barrett's is diagnosed early enough, it is possible to intervene before the disease progresses to cancer.

The fact that sometimes patients don't seek a medical diagnosis is critical. The incidence of one type of esophageal cancer, adenocarcinoma at the junction of the esophagus and stomach, has increased in percentage more than any other cancer in the world.

All of these facts made me very pleased to read Dr. Shekhar Challa's "Spurn the Burn." One of the most common requests from patients in my practice has been for more information about heartburn, hiatal hernias, Barrett's esophagus, and other related problems. It just wasn't available in a written format that the layperson could easily understand.

This book changes that. It serves a tremendous purpose in giving individuals access to solid, common sense information about heartburn, GERD, Barrett's Esophagus, esophageal cancer,

Foreword by Dr. Bergein Overholt

and the important aspects of treating this disease. It offers succinct information about treatment options — both the tried and true methods and newly emerging options.

Dr. Challa has done it again, producing a useful, informative book on a topic that affects millions of people in the United States. Now GERD patients will have the information they have been requesting — and needing.

Bergein Overholt, MD, FACP, MACG
Gastrointestinal Associates, PC
Knoxville, Tennessee

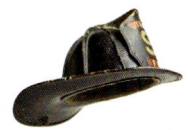

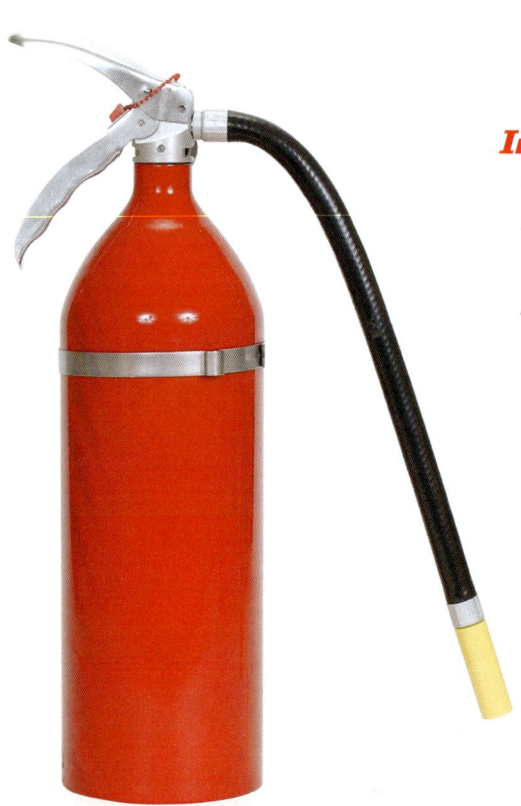

In this introduction…
- Heartburn vs. GERD
- The epidemic proportions of GERD
- The changing face of GERD diagnosis and treatment

Introduction

The Epidemic of a New Millennium

> *A man too busy to take care of his health is like a mechanic too busy to take care of his tools.*
> ~ Spanish proverb

GERD on the Rise

The sizzling fire of heartburn is a familiar sensation to millions of people. Sixty million Americans, to be exact. That many people report heartburn at least once a month, and 10 percent of the country's population is challenged with the condition daily.

Heartburn that occurs more than twice a week may be the indication of a medical condition called Gastroesophageal Reflux Disease, or GERD. (In Europe and other countries, the disease is referred to as GORD, because *esophageal* is spelled *oesophageal*.) Victims of this disease label it in a variety of ways, some correct and some not — acid reflux, heartburn, and even hiatal hernia.

The "simple" explanation of GERD is that stomach acid and other stomach contents come back up (reflux) into the esophagus (the food pipe) or the back of the throat. This is what causes many of the aggravating GERD symptoms highlighted in commercials and pharmaceutical advertisements such as heartburn, regurgitation, and burning sensation in the chest or throat.

Reflux occurs normally in everyone, but with GERD it is exaggerated, damaging the esophagus and potentially leading to more intense symptoms and serious consequences. If nothing else, GERD can make life miserable, forcing sufferers to give up favorite foods or to dread eating because it frequently results in discomfort and pain.

It is a chronic medical condition that can and usually does affect quality of life, interfering with daily activities. For some people, nighttime sleeping patterns are disrupted, too. In about 10 percent of patients, GERD leads to Barrett's esophagus, a pre-cancerous condition. Barrett's esophagus can in turn lead to esophageal cancer, which has a very poor prognosis.

Studies have shown that quality of life for people suffering from GERD is worse than for those who are ill with heart disease. 40 percent of patients report below normal functioning the day after they've dealt with a nocturnal GERD episode.

When quality of life is affected to that degree, GERD sufferers go looking for answers, and they look first at pharmacy shelves. The American public spends more than $10 billion annually on medications related to GERD.

For those battling the bulge (and most people are familiar with reports on the high rate of obesity in the United States), GERD is often a frustrating reality. The multiplying number of GERD cases is also reflected in the increase of esophageal cancer cases — up by 350 percent compared with twenty years ago. In

Introduction — The Epidemic of a New Millenium

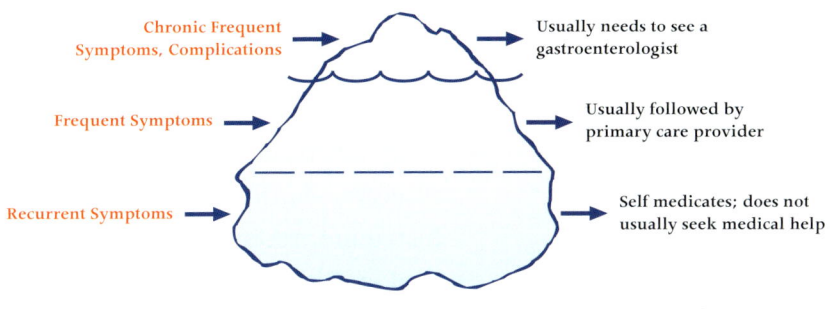

FIGURE 1. Iceberg Illustration

fact, compared with all other cancers, esophageal cancer is the most rapidly increasing cancer in the United States.

In most medical practices, physicians are seeing only the tip of the iceberg in problems related to GERD. The proliferation of over-the-counter medications available means that many people are choosing to treat their heartburn themselves, gulping down liquid antacids or popping tablets by the handful. Many view heartburn as a normal part of their lives, not even realizing the need to consult a doctor.

GERD sufferers may hesitate to seek help from their doctors due to misconceptions about procedures used to diagnose the disease. The word *endoscopy* is enough to send shudders through a patient and cause that acid to creep back up in the throat; the mere idea of inserting a tube through the mouth and down the throat can cause mental gagging.

Even health care personnel sometimes don't understand the purpose of an endoscopy, the most common procedure used to diagnose GERD. Although the disease frequently is diagnosed based on patient symptoms, an endoscopy is crucial to rule out

Spurn the Burn

> *I have suffered from acid reflux off and on for years. The past year, it has gotten so much worse, especially at night. I wasn't sleeping and so it was even interfering with work. But I put off going to my doctor because I figured he couldn't do much more for me than the over-the-counter medications could. I also didn't want to stick any tubes down my throat. Finally, though, I was so miserable that it was worth anything to get some relief, just to be able to lie down without feeling that acid creep back up my throat. Once I found out how simple diagnosis and treatment were, I couldn't believe I hadn't gone for help sooner. I can now sleep all night!*
>
> ~ Max, age 48

Barrett's esophagus and esophageal cancer.

Treatment options have dramatically advanced over the past twenty years, shuffling from antacids to histamine$_2$-receptor antagonists like Zantac, Tagamet, Axid, and Pepcid. Then in 1989, the first of a new class of medicines for GERD, called PPIs or proton pump inhibitors (the first was Prilosec), was approved by the Food and Drug Administration (FDA). Since that time, the list of PPIs has grown to include Prevacid, Aciphex, Protonix, Nexium, and Zegerid. They now are the best medicines available to fight GERD — just ask the many celebrities peppering the PPI advertisements in magazines and on television.

Few diseases destroy quality of life but are as easily treated as GERD. Patients have numerous options to change the way their lives are affected. The first crucial step is eliminating the possibility of serious, life-threatening problems. Then, with the help of this book and a medical professional, it is possible to significantly change the impact GERD has on one's daily life.

It is my desire to increase awareness of GERD and its complications and to help GERD sufferers gain an understanding of the

Introduction — The Epidemic of a New Millenium

huge strides being made in the diagnosis of this disease — specifically with the Bravo capsule and the PillCam. These new advances will help patients ease their anxieties, get the help they need, and spurn the burn.

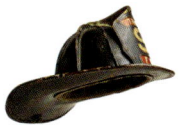

Spurn the Burn

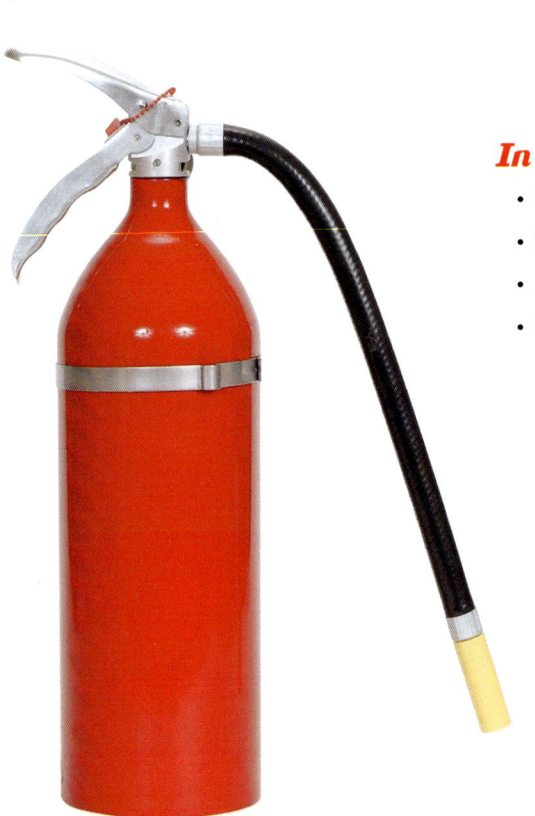

In this chapter...
- Charles Wurm
- Sue Michalski
- Jim Cline
- Carlene Parks

Chapter One
No Respecter of Persons

Health is not valued 'til sickness comes.
~ Thomas Fuller

Faces of GERD

Lack of sleep, discomfort, and the inability to eat favorite foods are just some of the challenges that individuals with GERD face on a daily basis. Surveys of these patients found they ranked their quality of life at a lower level than people with heart disease did.

GERD doesn't discriminate; it challenges people of all age groups and races, as well as both genders. What is assured is that GERD symptoms will change the life of anyone affected by the disease.

Charles Wurm

For most, as with Charles Wurm, age sixty-two, it is easy to ignore the symptoms at first.

Spurn the Burn

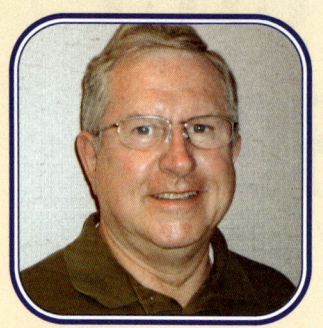

FIGURE 2
Charles Wurm, age 62

"It wouldn't go away," he said. "Then I used over-the-counter medicines, like Tums and Maalox and just tried to live my life by ignoring it."

Gradually, the symptoms of heartburn worsened. As a student late in life, studying at age fifty to be a physician's assistant, Charles began to learn more about GERD. He identified his own symptoms as acid reflux and began to become concerned.

"Eventually, things would get stuck in my throat and I would almost choke," he said. "But even this I was able to ignore."

That stubbornness eventually gave way as Charles experienced even more severe symptoms to the point that food was getting impacted in his esophagus and he knew he could have a serious problem.

Charles went to the doctor and had an endoscopy done.

It came back with bad news: Not only did he have severe acid reflux disease, but Charles was suffering from Barrett's esophagus, a pre-cancerous condition. But the good news was that, since the condition was diagnosed early enough, Charles and his physician could monitor closely and treat the situation. They have done this through periodic endoscopies and by Charles taking prescription medications.

He's also adjusted his diet, drinking coffee only in the morning and never at night. He doesn't eat within two hours of bedtime, a standard recommendation for people with GERD.

No Respecter of Persons

"I think it's a lifestyle disease in that I'm a little overweight and … I have a hiatal hernia, which is a consequence of that additional weight," Charles explained. "A significant number of people in America have hiatal hernias. With the epidemic of obesity in this country, that statistic is only going to grow. If you're overweight, you're prone to reflux. If you don't eat the right foods, you're prone to reflux. If you eat and lie down on the couch, you're more prone to reflux. In that regard, the modern American lifestyle makes people more prone to reflux."

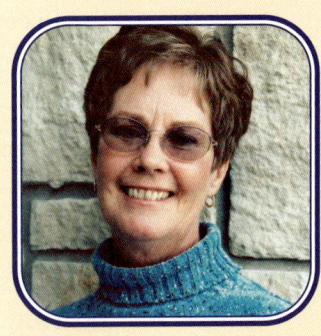

FIGURE 3
Sue Michalski, age 55

Sue Michalski

Sue Michalski, age fifty-five, completely understands Charles' willingness to ignore the initial symptoms. She was unsure what was happening when she was first hit with the disease about twelve years ago, and it seemed like a relatively mild problem.

"It was just a burning in my throat and I didn't know what it was," she said. "I went to a doctor and started with over-the-counter medications. I was eating Rolaids."

Like Charles, Sue found that her symptoms were worsening.

"I had a cough, and my chest was hurting," she recalled. "It was worse at night. I wasn't sleeping. I wasn't eating well. Actually, in an effort to absorb the acid, I started eating all these starchy foods. I'd think *I'll eat this and it will help absorb the acid*. Of course, then I gained weight."

Since the disease crept up on her in small increments, Sue said she wasn't immediately aware of how much it was affecting her life.

"I'd sleep sitting up," she said. "Or I'd have to lie a certain way to try to control the reflux. It seemed as if everything I ate bothered me — everything! I think if I could have controlled it by staying away from certain foods, it would have been easier."

While visiting with her doctor about something else, Sue mentioned the acid reflux and cough. He gave her a thirty-day trial of a prescription medication. It worked well for a while but then didn't seem to be as effective. Sue's doctor switched her to another medication, and then another one. She finally found one that worked for almost two years, Sue said.

But life was stressful at the time: Sue's father died and she began taking care of her mother, who was chronically ill. Being stressed exacerbated the symptoms, and Sue began self-medicating, doubling dosages of the medicines and adding over-the-counter heartburn and acid reflux medications to her daily routine.

More than a year ago, she woke up one morning and was in such pain that her husband was convinced she was having a heart attack. After a visit to the emergency room and heart tests that showed no problems, Sue knew that the acid reflux was out of control.

She underwent surgery just over a year ago, and that alleviated most of her symptoms. Occasionally, she'll have problems after eating particular foods or if she eats too near bedtime. But she is taking no medication now for GERD.

No Respecter of Persons

Jim Cline

Although Charles and Sue identified their problems almost immediately, GERD symptoms are not always that definitive. Jim Cline, age sixty-eight, began coughing all the time about three years ago.

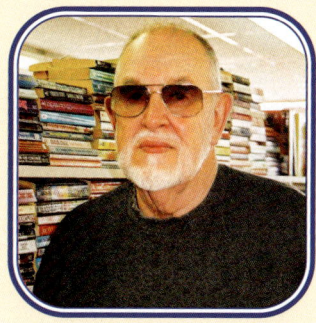

FIGURE 4
Jim Cline, age 68

"I had coughing fits where most of the day I'd just sit there and cough," he remembered.

Since a cough can fit so many different diagnoses, there began a time of trying to determine what was wrong. His physician assumed at first that he was suffering from allergies. But medications for that problem didn't help. The cough continued, and Jim was referred to a lung specialist, who ran numerous tests. Nothing definitive was found, and it was extremely frustrating.

"After I would have the coughing fits, I'd just be worn out," he said. "There were cold, clammy sweats. My throat was hurting from coughing so much."

Finally, Jim's physician referred him for an endoscopy and also talked about the possibility of doing a forty-eight-hour pH Bravo test, which would measure a variety of factors that indicate the presence and severity of the reflux. He was diagnosed with GERD and a hiatal hernia. Jim had surgery to repair the problem. Before the endoscopy, Jim said he wasn't familiar with acid reflux and had no idea that it could be causing his cough.

Spurn the Burn

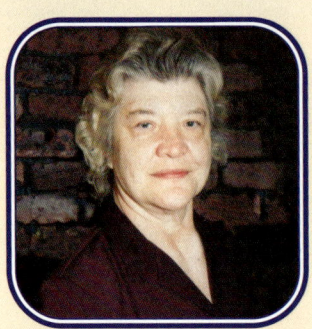

FIGURE 5
Carlene Parks, age 64

Carlene Parks

Coughing alone, without acid reflux or heartburn, is not the way GERD normally presents, which is why Jim's physicians didn't immediately consider the problem. GERD also can be masked by other illnesses, as in the case of Carlene Parks, age sixty-four. She had gallbladder problems and assumed that most of her symptoms were related to that condition.

Carlene was aware that she had occasional problems with acid reflux — bad enough that she sat up in the recliner to sleep some nights. She had also had a chronic cough, but dismissed that as part of some asthma-related problems with which she had struggled. Her physician began treating her with a prescription medication, which did not help tremendously. In the midst of dealing with GERD, she had gallbladder surgery. But based on the results of an endoscopy, her physician began to suspect the cough was GERD-related.

Considering her symptoms, which were not severe, Carlene was surprised to find that an endoscopy showed her as "one of the worst GERD patients I have ever seen," according to the physician who performed the procedure.

Carlene adjusted her diet to accommodate GERD, giving up pizza and tacos. "It's funny the way the disease can impact you," she said. She coughed so much that her three-year-old grandson began mimicking and still does so today.

No Respecter of Persons

"As soon as he would see me, he'd walk up and start coughing," she said.

As these cases illustrate, GERD or its complications can manifest itself with various symptoms, some typical and some atypical. There are no particular groups of people that suffer from this disease, and often there is no way to tell if one is a "candidate" for GERD. There are certain lifestyle and dietary choices (discussed in chapter 2, "Burn, Baby, Burn!") that can make a person more likely to suffer from some of the GERD symptoms, such as heartburn.

> **AUTHOR'S NOTE**
> I have been in practice for eighteen years, and the atypical symptoms are the toughest to diagnose without testing. Something like a cough can be caused by a wide variety of medical issues. One must be persistent in determining the cause of any ailment before dismissing it as "nothing serious."

The important point to remember is that you may begin successfully treating GERD symptoms with over-the-counter medications, but you still should consult a physician. As you will learn throughout this book, there are potentially life-threatening complications that can arise from acid reflux. Don't wait.

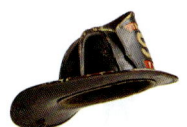

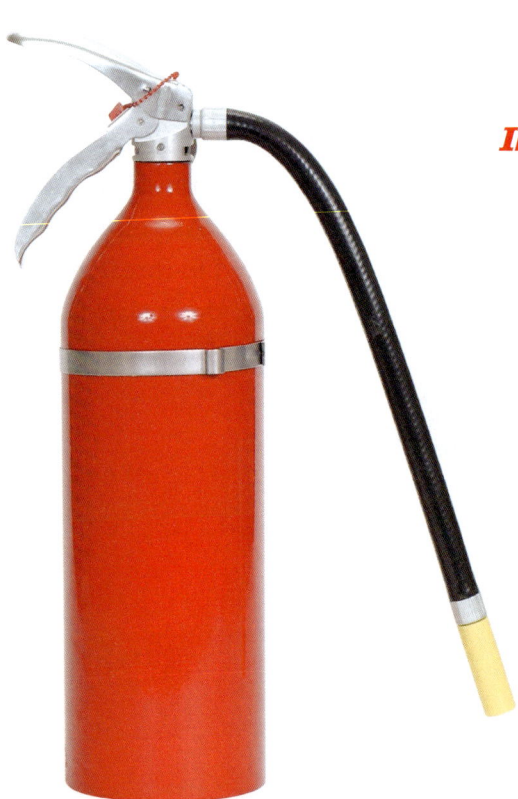

In this chapter...

- Typical and atypical symptoms of GERD
- Medications that aggravate GERD symptoms
- NERD vs. GERD

Chapter Two
Burn, Baby, Burn!

I would like to find a stew that will give me heartburn immediately, instead of at three o'clock in the morning.
~ John Barrymore

The Signs and Symptoms of GERD

Many a tale is told about people who thought they had heartburn but instead suffered heart attacks. Lewis, age fifty-seven, suffered from the opposite problem. He was awakened in the middle of the night with a tight pain in his chest. Panicked, he awakened his wife, sure he was having a heart attack. Three hours later, after an ambulance ride and numerous tests, he was released from the emergency room with a diagnosis that was both a relief and an embarrassment: GERD. GERD is well known for its most prominent symptom of heartburn. This painful problem is depicted frequently in advertisements that paint dramatic pictures of that tight, burning sensation in the center of the chest, which, as Lewis did, can easily be mistaken for a heart problem.

Although heartburn is indeed one of the symptoms of GERD,

COMMON (TYPICAL) SYMPTOMS OF GERD
- Heartburn
- Regurgitation
- Waterbrash (excess salivation)
- Dysphagia (difficulty swallowing)
- Odonophagia (pain with swallowing)
- Epigastric (upper abdominal) pain

UNCOMMON (ATYPICAL) SYMPTOMS OF GERD
- Chest pain
- Pulmonary or lung-related symptoms, such as chronic cough, asthma, recurrent bronchial infections
- Ear, nose, and throat symptoms, such as chronic laryngitis or hoarseness
- Dental erosions
- Globus (sensation of a lump in the throat) or a repeated feeling or need to clear one's throat
- Bad breath (halitosis)
- Belching
- Chronic sore throat

not everyone with the disease suffers from it. This complex disease has many manifestations. Most GERD symptoms probably are caused by hydrochloric acid, which is secreted by the parietal cells of the stomach, that comes back up into the esophagus. Each of us has some kind of gastroesophageal reflux on a daily basis, but it typically is not associated with symptoms like heartburn.

Most Common (Typical) GERD Symptoms

- **Heartburn** is by far the most common symptom of GERD. The sensation of burning in the upper chest starts just below the sternum and moves up into the throat. It is worse after meals, when one is bending over, and also at night (nocturnal reflux). Sixty million Americans experience heartburn monthly, twenty-five million have heartburn weekly, and thirteen million report heartburn as a daily occurrence. Be sure to describe your heartburn to the physician. It may mean a different symptom to a different person.

Burn, Baby, Burn!

- **Regurgitation** is described as the effortless return of acidic stomach contents from the stomach into the esophagus and throat.

- **Waterbrash** is the excess salivation that occurs in response to reflux.

- **Dysphagia and odonophagia** mean difficulty swallowing and painful swallowing, respectively. When GERD is progressive, these symptoms could be a sign of complications and should be considered a red flag. (See chapter 4, "What Went Wrong?" for more information).

- **Epigastric pain** is typically a pain or discomfort that is centered in the upper abdominal area. It can be a symptom of reflux in association with other symptoms or by itself.

- **Nocturnal reflux** may be one of the most frustrating, difficult parts of having GERD. Its name is self-explanatory: reflux that occurs when lying down at night. Reflux symptoms at night may be worse for several reasons. Normally gravity helps "push" stomach contents from the esophagus into the stomach. When in a horizontal position, you lose the advantage of gravity. During sleep, salivation decreases and you lose the neutralizing effects of the bicarbonate in saliva on the stomach acid. Esophageal

> *I've never forgotten the embarrassment of feeling my stomach contents come back up in my throat. It usually happened at night and I'd awaken suddenly, jerking up in bed and gasping, sometimes even spitting up. When I was dating my wife and she would stay over, I would worry about that happening in front of her.*
> ~ Walter, age 39

> *I was always fine during the day, but the minute I would lay down at night, I could feel the acid eating away at my throat. It would bubble up and I would end up sleeping in my husband's recliner. It was the only way I got any rest at all, and I still was exhausted constantly. It was so wonderful to start taking medicine — it means I can sleep in my bed at night!*
> ~ Marisha, age 48

peristalsis, the wavelike motion that pushes food through the esophagus, is decreased while sleeping. People don't experience heartburn during sleep, as this is a conscious, waking phenomenon. For this reason, sleep-related reflux episodes may last longer, even up to twenty minutes or more in some people.

Nocturnal symptoms of GERD can be one of the most disturbing aspects of the disease; they can have a dire effect on quality of life and can affect work productivity immensely. Up to 40 percent of the patients report "below normal" functioning the day after a nocturnal reflux episode. The quality of life scores in nighttime reflux show there is a significant decrease in both physical and mental components. There is enough evidence in the literature that complications of GERD are more severe in patients with nighttime symptoms of the disease. Those patients report such difficulties as trouble falling asleep, frequent awakening, and poor sleep quality. Going to bed within two hours of eating may worsen nocturnal reflux.

Less Common (Atypical) GERD Symptoms

- **Chest Pain** is one symptom that should be assumed to be caused by cardiac problems until proven otherwise. If you're having chest pains, the heart should be the first con-

Burn, Baby, Burn!

sideration. Having said that, it is not uncommon to have chest pain that is non-cardiac and may be connected to GERD. Time and again, gastrointestinal professionals receive referrals from cardiology peers after cardiac causes of the problem have been ruled out.

> Some patients cannot differentiate heartburn from chest pain and use these terms interchangeably. Some describe it as pressure, some say pain, whereas others refer to it as fullness. It is important that patients and physicians be aware of this and make sure they are on the same page when talking about this symptom.

- **Chronic cough, asthma, and repeated bronchial infections** can all be caused by GERD. Asthma can be a common manifestation of GERD in children. In addition, in children GERD could be a contributing factor in recurrent sinus and/or ear infections. The cause of asthma in at least 30 percent of patients (some studies say 70 percent) is secondary to GERD. Physicians must consider GERD as a causal factor if a patient develops asthma as an adult. Also, they should consider GERD as a cause of asthma if GERD symptoms get worse when patients are prescribed the asthma drug Theophylline, as this drug relaxes the lower esophageal sphincter — the opening between the esophagus and the stomach.

- **Dental decay** can be a symptom of GERD because acid reflux that reaches the mouth repeatedly can erode dental enamel, causing tooth decay.

- **Other symptoms** such as the sensation of needing to clear your throat, lump in the throat sensation, hiccups, bad

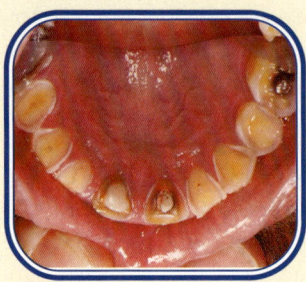

FIGURE 6
Dental decay

~

Sleep apnea is sometimes connected with GERD, but the relationship between the two is actually unclear. Scientific studies have shown that even though both conditions have similar risk factors, there might not be a true relationship between the two.

breath, chronic laryngitis, hoarseness, belching, and chronic sore throat can all be indicative of GERD.

Physicians and patients should be familiar with the atypical symptoms and aware of the possibility of GERD whenever such symptoms occur.

Two Kinds of Reflux Disease

Based on an endoscopy, a procedure that enables physicians to examine the esophagus, patients with GERD can be divided into two basic categories: erosive esophagitis (30 percent) or non-erosive reflux disease (70 percent).

Erosive esophagitis means that there is evidence of injury to the esophagus, typically caused by GERD. Based on the severity, it is graded on a scale of 1 (the least injury) to 4 (the most injury) or from A to D, depending on the system the physician uses.

Non-erosive reflux disease (NERD) means the patient shows no evidence of any mucosal injury to the esophagus. But just because there is no evidence of injury does not mean the person has a mild version of GERD. In fact, patients with NERD may need higher doses of medicine to treat the condition than patients with esophagitis. It is one of the paradoxes of the disease.

Burn, Baby, Burn!

Given this list of symptoms and signs, it is clear that GERD can have a terrible impact on anyone's quality of life.

Other Factors that May Aggravate GERD Symptoms

One of the frustrating things for those suffering from GERD is that different lifestyle factors and dietary choices aggravate the symptoms in each person. However, to follow is a list of things that tend to exacerbate GERD in most people:

- Gaining weight (pregnancy, obesity)
- Chocolate
- Caffeine in coffee, tea, or cola drinks
- Alcohol
- Peppermint
- Citrus juices
- Tomato products
- Spicy foods
- Raw onions
- Fatty foods
- Smoking
- Hiatal hernia

Medications that May Aggravate GERD Symptoms

There are several medications that can aggravate GERD. Some of these medications

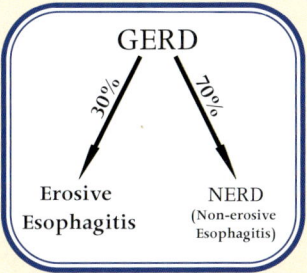

FIGURE 7
NERD & GERD

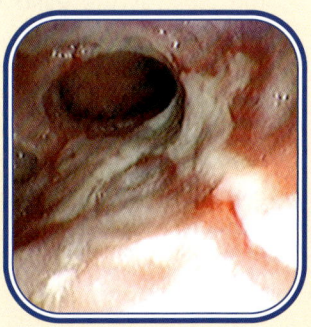

FIGURE 8
Esophagitis

The mucosa is the innermost layer of the gastrointestinal tract. In different areas of the gastrointestinal tract, the mucosa is composed of different types of cells. In the esophagus, these cells are called squamous cells, and in the stomach, they are called columnar cells.

There need not be a correlation between severity of symptoms and severity of findings in GERD when an endoscopy is done. Some people with severe symptoms will have a normal endoscopy and other with minimal symptoms may be found to have severe esophagitis. It is indeed a humbling experience for even the most astute gastroenterologists to attempt to guess the severity of findings based on symptoms alone, as they frequently will find out how wrong they can be. That is why it's so important that patients be tested.

cause the opening between the esophagus (the tube the food goes down) and the stomach to relax; others slow down the movement of food through the esophagus; and still others cause damage to the lining of the esophagus.

These medications include the following:

- Beta$_2$ agonists (salbutamol [Ventolin, Volmax] and terbutaline [Bricanyl])
- NSAIDs (e.g., aspirin, Motrin, Naprosyn)
- Theophylline
- Calcium channel blockers (e.g., Norvasc, Cardizem, Procardia)
- Beta blockers (Inderal and Tenormin)
- Anti-Parkinson's medications (Levodopa)
- Birth control pills
- Anti-cholinergic medications
- Tricyclic antidepressants (Elavil and Tofranil)
- Sedatives (e.g., Valium)
- Narcotics (e.g., Demerol)
- Bone-density medications (e.g., Fosamax)

As evident in this chapter, the signs of GERD are not always the obvious to the patient and sometimes are not even evident to the physician. Heartburn, of course, is the most recognized symp-

Burn, Baby, Burn!

tom, but it is important to remember that some of the less-frequent symptoms discussed here can be a sign of GERD. Becoming familiar with your own personal signs and symptoms, as well as the aggravating factors that heighten those symptoms, can go a long way toward improving your quality of life.

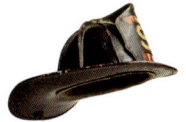

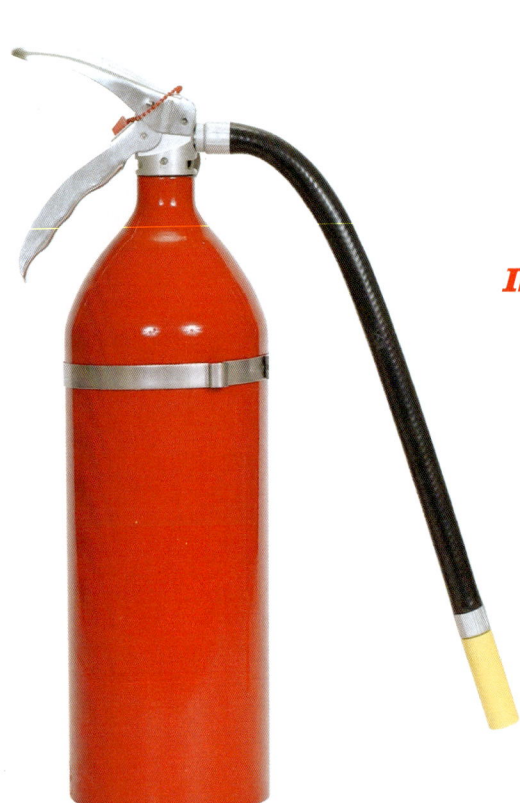

In this chapter...
- The normal digestive process
- Malfunction of the LES
- Hiatal Hernia and GERD

Chapter Three
The Throat Bone's Connected to the Stomach Bone

It is easier to find men who will volunteer to die than to find those who are willing to endure pain with patience.
— Julius Caesar

The Anatomy of GERD

Whether it's a steak, an apple, or a slice of pizza, the food we eat follows a particular path through the body. The digestive system, or gastrointestinal tract, that makes this possible consists of the mouth, pharynx, esophagus, stomach, small intestine, large intestine (colon and rectum), and anus.

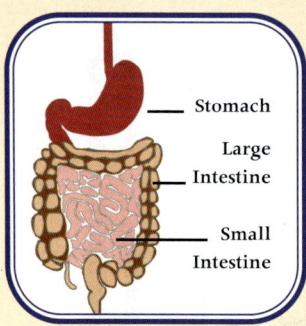

Figure 9
Digestive System

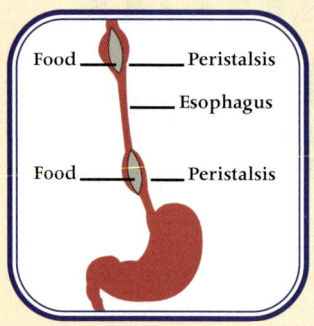

Figure 10
Peristalsis

Spurn the Burn

The Normal Digestive Process

When food is swallowed, it is moved through the digestive system by a process called peristalsis. As food comes in contact with the gastrointestinal tract, muscles contract, and in a wavelike manner, the food is propelled forward.

The esophagus — or food pipe — transports food from the throat to the stomach. It is eighteen to twenty-five centimeters in length and about seventeen millimeters in diameter. This hollow muscular tube has a valve (opening) at both ends called the upper and lower esophageal sphincters. After food enters the stomach, hydrochloric acid and other digestive enzymes break it down into small particles. The stomach produces an average of two liters of acid daily. The sight, smell, and taste of food and the presence of food in the stomach stimulate the secretion of this acid by the parietal cells in the stomach. The vagus nerve causes acid secretion through three pathways: the acetylcholine, gastrin, and histamine receptor pathways. (The effects of this acid secretion on GERD are explained in detail in chapter 6, "Pills, Knife, or No More Spice.")

After the food is pulverized in the stomach, it then is pushed

The Throat Bone's Connected to the Stomach Bone

into the small intestine through an opening at the base of the stomach called the pylorus. The small food particles are digested here in the small intestines, and all benefits and nutrients are absorbed at this point of digestion. Whatever is left after this process is complete is known as the waste, and it enters the colon (the large intestine). Most of the water from this waste is absorbed in the colon, and the remainder, the fecal matter, is eliminated through bowel movements through the rectum and anus.

Most of the esophagus is located in the chest. The diaphragm separates the chest and the abdominal cavity, and an opening in the right side, called the diaphragmatic hiatus, is where the esophagus enters the stomach. The lower esophageal sphincter (LES), a two- to four-centimeter muscle that acts like a valve, is located where the esophagus enters the stomach. This muscle works like a rubber band and holds the tube closed, preventing gastric contents from "refluxing" back up into the esophagus.

The LES is contracted even at rest, maintaining a pressure of between twelve and twenty millimeters of pressure, which is higher than the pressure in the stomach. When swallowing occurs, peristalsis begins at the esophagus, pushing the food

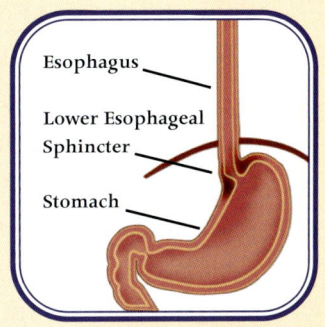

FIGURE 11
LES

~

The LES works like a trap door, allowing food to travel into the stomach, and if working properly, it closes to keep the stomach contents from coming back up into the esophagus.

through the food pipe and toward the lower esophageal sphincter, which then relaxes and allows food to enter the stomach.

Connecting the diaphragm and the LES is the phrenicoesophageal ligament. Its job is to keep the LES in the diaphragmatic hiatus. The LES, the diaphragm, and the phrenicoesophageal ligament make up the primary anti-reflux barrier.

GERD most often results from the "malfunction" of the LES. One way this happens is through something called TLESRs, an abbreviation for transient lower esophageal sphincter relaxation. This transient relaxation of the LES happens in everyone, most often after eating, to release swallowed air or gas in the stomach. Normally, a swallow relaxes the sphincter, usually for about five seconds. But in patients with GERD, TLESRs cause acid reflux. In this situation, they often are not associated with a swallow and may last up to thirty seconds.

So as explained here, the body has several built-in defenses to fight reflux: the anti-reflux mechanism involving the LES, the diaphragm, and the phrenicoesophageal ligament. If despite these defenses, reflux does occur, there are several secondary defenses that combat the reflux, including saliva to neutralize the acid, as well as gravity and peristalsis to push the acid down, decreasing the "contact time" of the acid to the esophagus wall.

Other Contributing Factors

- **Hypotensive LES:** This occurs in 20 percent of GERD patients and means the sphincter pressure is decreased, allowing the free flow of acid into the esophagus. Things like

The Throat Bone's Connected to the Stomach Bone

chocolate, alcohol, and peppermint decrease LES pressure. Some medications, including calcium channel blockers, nitrates, and theophylline, also decrease that pressure.

> *It is not uncommon for people to chew gum to combat [reflux] symptoms. It seems to work because it increases salivary production. The bicarbonate in saliva neutralizes acid. Gum also increases peristalsis.*
> *~ Dr. Jerry Feagan, gastroenterologist*

- **Anatomical distortion of the anti-reflux barrier:** This could happen if the patient has a hiatal hernia, as described in the following section.

- **Delayed gastric (stomach) emptying:** In approximately ten to 15 percent of GERD patients, there is a delay in the emptying of contents from the stomach — a problem that occurs sometimes with conditions like diabetes. This contributes to acid reflux due to stomach distension.

- **Delayed esophageal clearance:** This occurs when there is decreased esophageal motility, leading to delayed clearance of acid from the esophagus. This can occur in conditions like scleroderma and multiple sclerosis.

- **Decreased salivary production:** This occurs less frequently than the other problems listed here. The presence of bicarbonate in saliva gives it an acid neutralizing capacity. Decreased salivary production can occur in people who smoke.

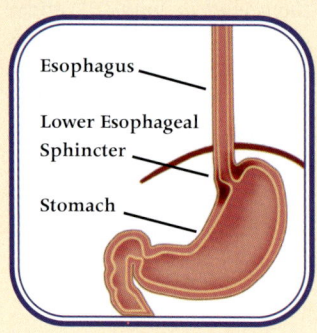

FIGURE 12A
Normal Anatomy

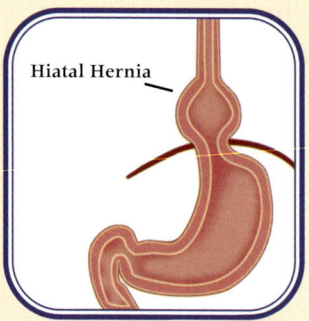

FIGURE 12B
Hiatal Hernia

- **Tissue resistance of esophageal mucosa:** Normally, esophageal mucosa has some ability to resist stomach acid. In some elderly or malnourished individuals, this can be decreased.

- **Increased intra-abdominal pressure:** This usually is associated with obesity and pregnancy and occurs when pressure is placed on the stomach.

- **Nighttime challenges:** Many people will notice that acid reflux seems to worsen at night. This may be because salivation is decreased while sleeping, esophageal motility is decreased, and lying flat on your back means gravity isn't helping.

Hiatal Hernia

One condition that needs special mention is a hiatal hernia. This term is sometimes erroneously used as an alternative for the terms *heartburn* or GERD. What it actually refers to is a medical condition in which part of the upper stomach goes through the hiatus of the diaphragm into the chest. This causes the di-

The Throat Bone's Connected to the Stomach Bone

aphragm to separate from the lower esophageal sphincter. In normal conditions, the diaphragm helps the sphincter by forming a firmer anti-reflux barrier. When a hiatal hernia forms, it may lead to a disruption of the primary defensive mechanism because of loss of the diaphragmatic support. That, in turn, leads to sphincter incompetence, which causes GERD. In addition, acid may be trapped in the hiatal hernia pouch, acting as a reservoir and causing reflux because it is located so close to the sphincter.

> *When I was a boy, my dad would always say, 'My hiatal hernia is acting up.' It was usually after he ate a big meal and he would rub the center of his chest. I thought hiatal hernia was synonymous with GERD until my doctor explained otherwise.*
>
> —Joe, age 72

It is unclear whether the hiatal hernia itself is an initiating factor in GERD, but if a person has GERD, the presence of a hiatal hernia makes it worse. Acts of straining and lifting, as well as obesity and pregnancy, can cause a hiatal hernia. But remember, one can have a hiatal hernia and not have GERD.

Many people will find they can simply treat their GERD symptoms with over-the-counter or prescription medications, without ever knowing exactly why they suffer from this disease. Determining the root of what is causing GERD, however, can be of primary importance in deciding how a patient should be treated if intervention beyond medication is required.

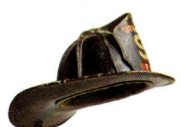

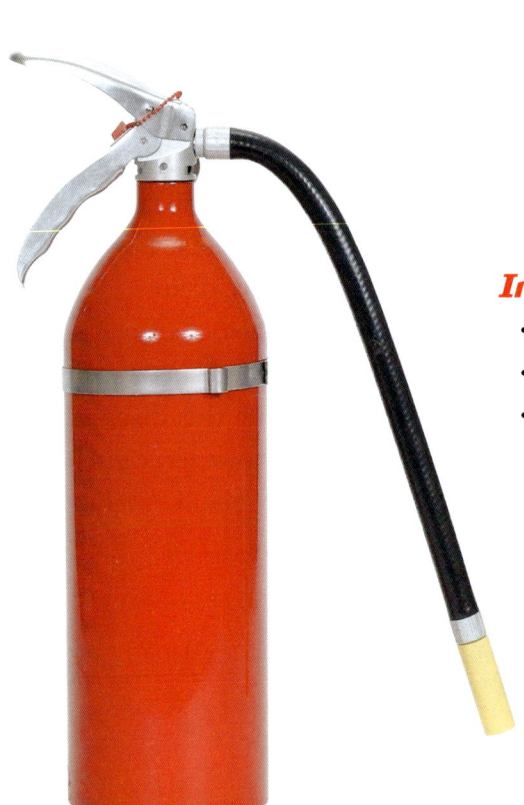

In this chapter...
- Barrett's esophagus
- Esophageal stricture
- Esophageal cancer

Chapter Four
What Went Wrong?

I treated my heartburn and reflux first by ignoring it. It wouldn't go away. Then I used over-the-counter medicines like Tums and Maalox. When I went to a doctor and had an endoscopy, I found that I had severe reflux disease. In fact, I had Barrett's esophagus, which is a precursor to esophageal cancer. That was really scary.
~ Charles Wurm

The Complications of GERD

Many people think that GERD is a relatively minor problem that can be treated with medication. For most people, that is an accurate assessment. But in a minority of patients, complications do develop, and some of those can have serious consequences.

GERD complications basically are the result of damage to the esophagus from repeated exposure to acid and other gastric juices. These problems need not correlate with the severity of the symptoms. In other words, a patient can have severe symptoms and not have complications, or a patient may have few or no symptoms but have severe complications.

Spurn the Burn

GERD COMPLICATIONS
- Erosive or ulcerative esophagitis
- Barrett's esophagus
- Esophageal stricture
- Esophageal adenocarcinoma (cancer)

~

When I went to the hospital, I was scared to death because I was throwing up blood. I was told I had ulcers in my esophagus. Thank goodness, they have now healed after taking medication.

— Sylvia, age 55

Erosive or Ulcerative Esophagitis

Esophageal inflammation caused by GERD is called reflux esophagitis. Don't forget, if you have GERD but there is no visible damage to the esophagus, you have NERD — non-erosive reflux disease. Patients who have NERD rarely progress to erosive esophagitis; once a NERD, always a NERD!

Patients with severe inflammation of the esophagus can develop erosions (mucosal breaks or "mini-ulcers" that are smaller and not as deep as ulcers) and/or ulcers. This can cause anemia from slow blood loss or on occasion can cause severe hemorrhage. As discussed in chapter 3, "The Throat Bone's Connected to the Stomach Bone," physicians grade the severity of the erosions on a scale of one (the least severe injury) to four (the most severe injury). Some doctors use A to D, but the essence of the grading is the same.

Barrett's Esophagus

Barrett's esophagus is a complication of long-standing, untreated GERD and is pre-malignant (pre-cancerous). Like erosive esophagitis, Barrett's esophagus is more common in men and in Caucasians. Also, the older the patient, the higher chance of

What Went Wrong?

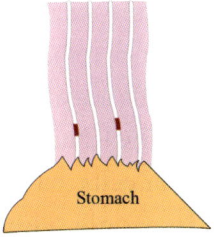

GRADE A
Small mucosal breaks of less than 5 mm.

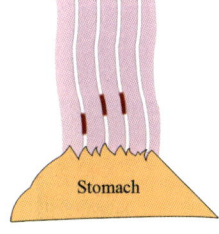

GRADE B
Small mucosal breaks of more than 5 mm.

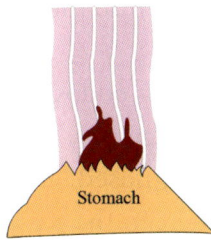

GRADE C
Mucosal breaks continue between folds but less than 75% of circumference.

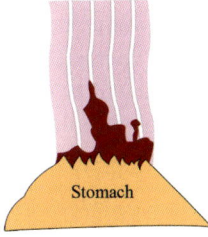

GRADE D
Mucosal breaks involving more than 75% of circumference.

FIGURE 13. Graded illustrations of esophagitis

being diagnosed with this complication. It is estimated that about 1.5 million Americans have Barrett's esophagus.

Between 10 and 20 percent of patients with GERD develop Barrett's esophagus. The longer you have GERD, the higher the chance that Barrett's will occur. In some patients, it can progress to dysplasia (pre-cancerous tissue changes). As you can see, the progression can occur in stages and should be monitored.

The esophagus lining is normally made of squamous cells,

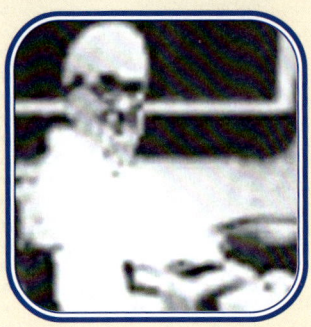

FIGURE 14
Barrett's esophagus was named after a British surgeon, Norman Rupert Barrett, who discovered the condition in 1950. (Photo courtesy of The Barrett's Oesophagus Foundation, England)

and the stomach and small intestine are lined with columnar cells. Over time, as the squamous cells are affected by the stomach acids, they change into specialized columnar cells that are not normally found in people. This change is called Barrett's esophagus. During an endoscopy, it appears as if there are tonguelike projections of salmon pink stomach coming into the pearly white esophagus.

If suspected at endoscopy, Barrett's must be confirmed by biopsy. After Barrett's is diagnosed, the physician will need to screen the patient periodically for the worsening of this pre-cancerous condition into dysplasia, an even more severe form of pre-cancerous cells. Dysplasia is categorized into low-grade (indicating pre-cancerous change of cells) or high-grade (indicating severe pre-cancerous change of cells). The frequency of these checks varies depending on the individual's situation. Visit with your doctor to determine a schedule.

There are no specific symptoms for Barrett's esophagus. Actually, patients who have Barrett's may have fewer symptoms, as the columnar cells that line the esophagus in this stage of the disease are more acid-resistant.

It is unclear why some people develop this complication and some don't. It does appear that increasing age, Caucasian background, and long-standing, untreated GERD are risk factors. In

What Went Wrong?

addition, there is a high incidence of Barrett's in patients with a hiatal hernia; in fact, the incidence increases with the size of the hernia.

The longer the duration of GERD symptoms, the higher the chance of developing Barrett's esophagus. In patients who have had symptoms for less than a year, there is less than a 5 percent chance of having Barrett's; symptoms for one to five years, a 10 percent chance of developing the complication; five to ten years of symptoms find 15 percent of patients with Barrett's; and patients with symptoms for more than ten years have a 20 percent incidence of Barrett's.

The treatment of Barrett's esophagus is essentially the same as treatment of GERD. Barrett's esophagus patients must be treated aggressively with PPIs (see chapter 6, "Pills, Knife, or No More Spice") regardless of the severity of symptoms. There is some evidence that if physicians treat GERD and Barrett's esophagus aggressively with long-standing medical therapy, the incidence of dysplasia is decreased. If dysplasia is found, however, the patient must be followed even more closely, and the physician may recommend surgery. There are some centers in the United States doing special procedures with an

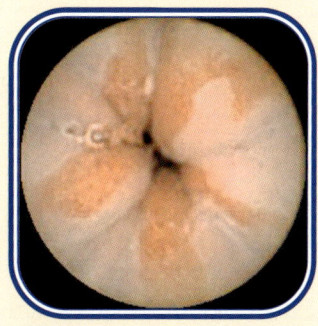

FIGURE 15A
Barrett's esophagus

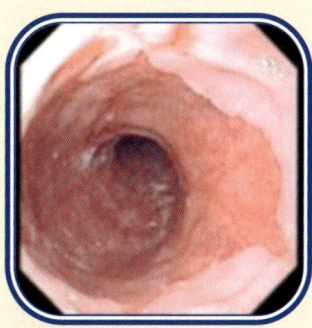

FIGURE 15B
Barrett's esophagus

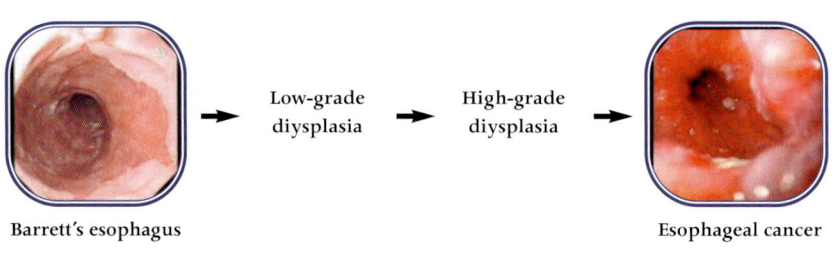

FIGURE 16: Progression from Barrett's esophagus to esophageal cancer

endoscope to treat dysplasia or very early cancer in Barrett's patients, especially if they are high risk for surgery. Possible procedures include photodynamic therapy (PDT) and endoscopic mucosal resection, although most insurance companies still have these labeled as "experimental."

A few centers in the United States perform PDT. During this procedure, a photosensitizing drug (called porfimer sodium) is injected intravenously. This drug stays in cancer cells longer than in other cells. Twenty-four to seventy-two hours later, the cancer cells in the esophagus are exposed to light through an endoscope, which activates the photosensitizer. When those photosensitizers are exposed to a particular wavelength of light, they emit oxygen, which kills nearby cells. In this case, the cancer cells are targeted.

Endoscopic mucosal resection is done with an endoscope, again in only a few centers in the United States. This is reserved for Barrett's esophagus with high-grade dysplasia or very early cancer. The specialist injects under the lesion, thereby lifting it, and the lesion is then "resected" with a snare, which lassoes the area. If esophageal surgery is needed, it is a major surgery and

What Went Wrong?

beyond the scope of this book to discuss in detail. A physician can provide further information.

It is expected that the PillCam, a new tool available to physicians to look at the inside of the esophagus, will dramatically increase the number of people getting screened for Barrett's, as it is noninvasive. (This new technology is explained in detail in chapter 5, "Open Up and Say, 'Ah!'")

Esophageal Stricture

Patients with long-standing GERD can develop narrowing of the esophagus, or esophageal stricture. GERD is the most common cause of esophageal stricture and about 85 percent of patients with stricture also have a hiatal hernia. This usually occurs at the gastroesophageal junction, which, as the name implies, is where the esophagus ends and the stomach begins.

> Mandatory screening guidelines for Barrett's esophagus include any patients who have had GERD symptoms for more than five years, male patients, Caucasian patients, and older patients (more than 40 years), regardless of the severity of symptoms. With Barrett's esophagus, the columnar epithelium shows decreased sensitivity to refluxed acid, which is why physicians cannot rely on symptoms to predict Barrett's. Moreover, even if the patient has symptoms that resolve with treatment, it is possible he or she may still have Barrett's esophagus.
>
> Every patient with long-standing GERD symptoms should be checked for Barrett's esophagus by endoscopy or the new non-invasive modality, the PillCam ESO (see chapter 5, "Open Up and Say, 'Ah!'").

Constant and repeated acid damage of the esophagus can lead to inflammation, erosions (mucosal breaks), and ulcers. When ulcers heal, scar tissue can form and this might contract, causing narrowing or stricture formation. Patients with strictures may experience difficulty swallowing, especially solid foods, a condition called dysphagia. Occasionally, patients may have

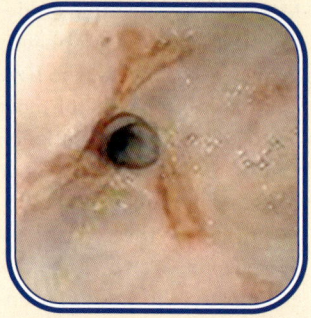

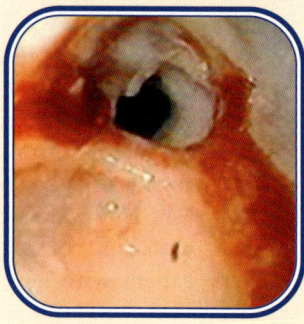

FIGURE 17
Esophageal stricture

~

As a truck driver, I'm on the road all the time. I'd been having some trouble swallowing but I was ignoring the problem and had just learned to chew my food well. But a few months ago, I was in Georgia on a run and ended up in the emergency room. The doctor called it food impaction. That scared me into seeking help for the stricture in my esophagus and now I get it stretched whenever I need to.

— Jeffrey, age 40

odonophagia, or painful swallowing. If a patient with these symptoms does not get checked, they sometimes may have food impacted above the stricture and may need an emergency endoscopic procedure for removal of that food. Strictures are treated with esophageal dilatation, in which dilators or a balloon is part of the endoscopic procedure. As scar tissue can be "elastic," patients do need repeated dilatation if and when difficulty swallowing reoccurs. Treatment of GERD with proton pump inhibitors will decrease the recurrence of esophageal strictures.

Esophageal Adenocarcinoma (Cancer of the Esophagus)

Cancer of the esophagus is one of the most lethal cancers of which the medical field is aware. The incidence of adenocarcinoma of the esophagus has risen by 350 percent over the past twenty years, more than any other type of cancer. The reason for this is unclear but it is believed to be caused by the increase in GERD.

Esophageal adenocarcinoma is more common in Caucasian men. Between

What Went Wrong?

twelve and thirteen thousand esophageal cancer cases are diagnosed in the United States annually, and 1 – 2 percent of patients per year with Barrett's esophagus develop esophageal adenocarcinoma. If you have Barrett's esophagus, your chance of getting adenocarcinoma is 40 to 125 times more likely than the general population.

Esophageal cancer is one of the most lethal cancers and the survival rate in esophageal adenocarcinoma over five years is only 10 percent. That's why it is particularly important to screen patients with Barrett's esophagus closely.

If a patient with GERD develops any alarming symptoms like anemia, weight loss, dysphagia, or persistent vomiting, concern should be raised immediately about esophageal adenocarcinoma. If the cancer is discovered very, very early, treatment is often surgical. Photodynamic therapy and endoscopic mucosal resection are also possibilities, although the availability of these procedures is limited to the few centers in the United States that perform them.

Overall prognosis for esophageal cancer is very poor, as most

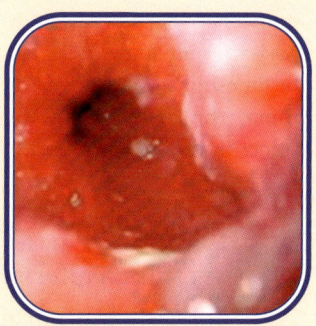

FIGURE 18
Cancer

~

I had problems with heartburn for twenty years. I treated it with lots and lots of Tums. When I started losing weight and began to have trouble swallowing, though, I went to the doctor, never dreaming the two things would be connected. I found out that I have cancer. Sometimes I wonder if I had gone in earlier, maybe they would have found it earlier and my prognosis would be more certain. Hindsight is 20/20.
~ Kalia, age 57

> Remember, Barrett's esophagus is the only known risk factor for esophageal adenocarcinoma, the fastest growing cancer in the western world.

of the time, when the diagnosis is made, the cancer has already moved outside the esophagus (metastasized).

Uncomfortable but Harmless or Deadly Serious?

As this chapter indicates, a disease that many consider uncomfortable but harmless can have serious complications. It is important to stress again that the severity of symptoms may not correlate with the severity of GERD and its complications. Any GERD symptoms should be perceived as potentially serious. Get checked by a doctor.

The complications of esophagitis, esophageal ulcers, bleeding, and stricture can be prevented or decreased by treating GERD aggressively with medications, but the complication of Barrett's esophagus and its pre-malignant potential cannot be decreased. The medical community is becoming increasingly aware of the higher incidence of esophageal cancer and how important it is to watch GERD patients, especially those who develop any of the alarming symptoms.

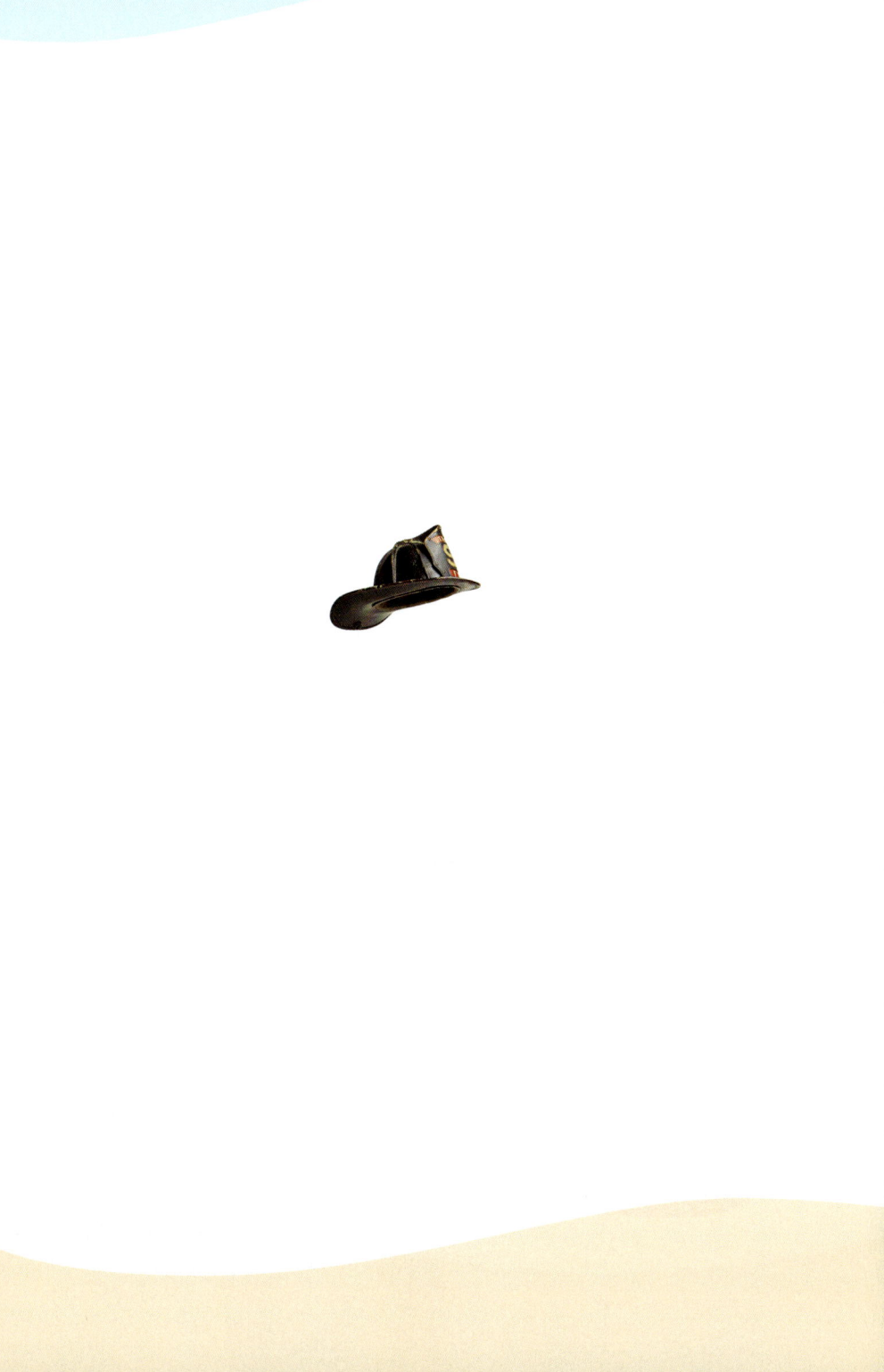

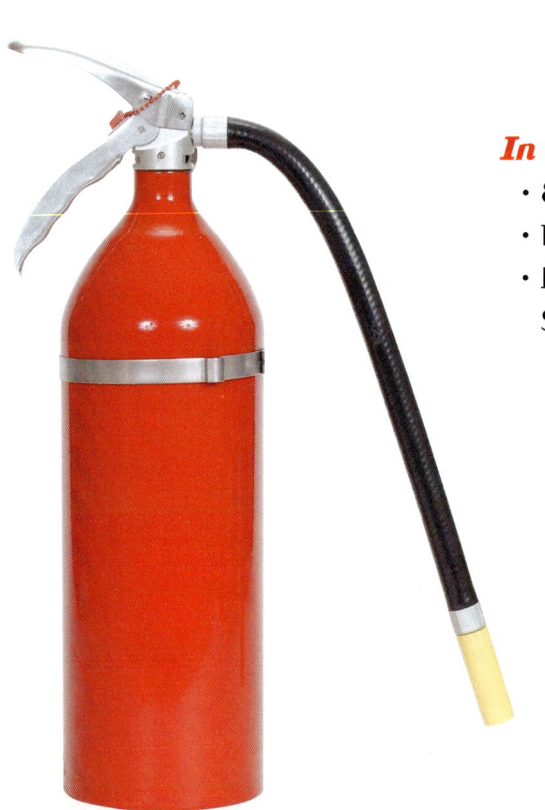

In this chapter...
- Endoscopy (EGD)
- PillCam ESO
- Bravo pH Monitoring System

Chapter Five
Open Up and Say, "Ah!"

Indigestion is the failure to adjust a square meal to a round stomach.
~ Anonymous

The Diagnosis of GERD

The symptoms of GERD are so well known to the general public that many patients often diagnose themselves and begin taking over-the-counter medications for heartburn and acid reflux. From the perspective of many physicians, these classic symptoms and a positive response to such medicines are all the evidence necessary to make a clinical diagnosis of GERD.

Why, then, is it necessary to do any tests at all? The answer is simple: Your doctor needs to make sure you do not have any complications of GERD, especially the pre-cancerous condition, Barrett's esophagus. Moreover, testing can reveal information that will help your doctor decide whether you need to be on medication all the time, regardless of symptoms, or whether you can take medication on an as-needed basis.

A vast majority of gastroenterologists are of the opinion patients should be checked at least once either with an endoscope or the new PillCam ESO if they have chronic symptoms of GERD. This is to rule out Barrett's esophagus. This is important because even if the patient's symptoms have disappeared upon treatment with medications, there is the possibility they may have this pre-cancerous condition.

~

Among the millions of people with GERD, it is estimated only 15 percent seek medical treatment. Remember the concept of the iceberg? It is my hope that the PillCam will encourage more patients to get checked as it involves just swallowing a capsule.

It is even more important to be tested if you have any of the alarming symptoms of weight loss, difficulty or pain with swallowing, blood in stool, anemia, or vomiting. The physician must determine whether GERD is causing these symptoms or if there are other complications.

Another reason your doctor may choose to proceed with tests is if you do not respond to treatment and/or you have atypical symptoms.

The primary test used to determine the condition of the esophagus and the effects of GERD is an EGD, or esophagogastroduodenoscopy. This is often simply referred to as an *endoscopy*. The PillCam, a recent entry into the field, may encourage GERD sufferers who have been uncomfortable seeking medical treatment to go in for testing. Forty-eight-hour esophageal pH with the Bravo pH Monitoring System is another test used for diagnosis.

Depending on the patient's symptoms, a physician may want to use one of these tests — an EGD, the PillCam ESO, or the Bravo pH Monitoring System. The test most commonly used today is the EGD. With its recent FDA approval, the PillCam may take over as the most popular test to diagnose GERD during the next few years. The forty-eight-hour Bravo pH test is used in situations

Open Up and Say, "Ah!"

in which the diagnosis is unclear, the physician needs to determine the severity of the reflux, or the patient is being prepared for surgery.

Esophagogastroduodenoscopy or EGD

During an EGD, the physician is able to examine the condition of the patient's esophagus, stomach, and duodenum (the beginning portion of the small intestines) using an instrument called a gastroscope. This flexible, lighted instrument passes through the patient's mouth via the throat into the esophagus, then the stomach, and finally into the duodenum. The patient is sedated for the procedure, and most people do not remember it when they awaken. The gastroscope is like an eye at the end of a long finger, and the physician can watch on a television screen to assess any possible damage from GERD. For an experienced physician, this procedure is just like driving a car. There are several knobs on the instrument through which the physician can maneuver through the esophagus, stomach, and duodenum. If an abnormality like Barrett's esophagus is found, the physician can take biopsies right then, which can be sent to the pathologist immediately.

An EGD is not painful because the patient is sedated, and it

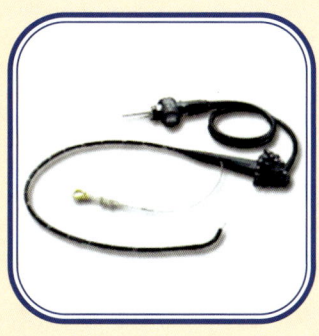

FIGURE 19
Gastroscope

~

I lost sleep the night before my EGD, dreading it even though my doctor said it wasn't a big deal. She was right. I was sedated and don't even remember the procedure. What's more, it laid my mind at rest about having cancer.
—Carmen, age 33

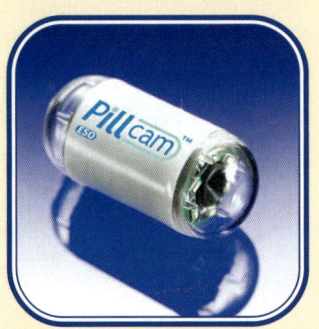

FIGURE 20
PillCam ESO

takes anywhere from ten to twenty minutes to complete. Complications, such as perforation or bleeding, are very rare. If you are on blood-thinning agents like Coumadin, aspirin, or Plavix, be sure to visit with your doctor about whether you should stop those medications prior to having this procedure done. Also, it's important to inform your doctor if you have an artificial heart valve or a prosthesis of any kind as this may require administration of antibiotics prior to the procedure. Diabetic patients on oral medications or insulin may be told to decrease or hold the medication prior to procedure.

Remember, the severity of the symptoms the patient is experiencing does not necessarily correlate with the findings from an EGD.

PillCam ESO

The PillCam ESO video capsule was approved by the FDA in October 2004. This new technology may very well change the way that physicians diagnose GERD and check for potential complications. It is a convenient, safe, and noninvasive way to screen patients with GERD to determine if they have Barrett's esophagus.

PillCam ESO is just what the name implies: a video camera inside a capsule pill that is the size of an average vitamin pill. It is swallowed by the patient with a sip of water and takes only a few minutes to traverse the esophagus. During that short jour-

Open Up and Say, "Ah!"

ney, the video camera captures images at the rate of fourteen frames per second. Those images are transmitted to a data recorder and are then uploaded to a computer and reviewed by the physician. The PillCam has a battery life of thirty minutes and is excreted in the stool.

If the PillCam shows any evidence of Barrett's esophagus or any other pathology, the physician will need to perform an EGD to confirm the diagnosis with a biopsy.

Most patients with GERD symptoms do not seek medical attention, especially if their symptoms are improved by over-the-counter medications. (Remember the iceberg concept!) Therefore, they are not being screened for Barrett's esophagus. There are several reasons this is happening, but the primary one is lack of information. Patients often don't understand that in a certain number of GERD cases, pre-cancerous conditions can develop. For some people, it is the fear of endoscopy that keeps them from seeking help.

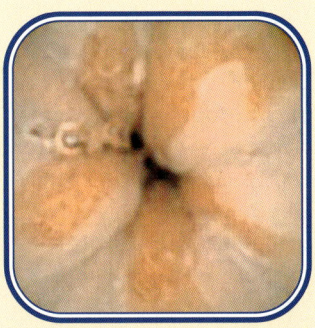

FIGURE 21A
PillCam picture of Barrett's Esophagus

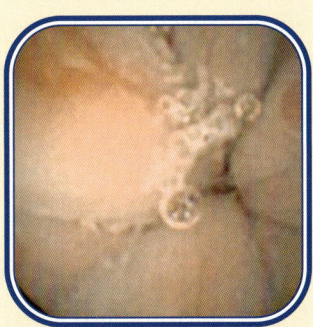

FIGURE 21B
PillCam picture of esophagitis

The PillCam ESO might revolutionize the screening of GERD patients, as it removes the fear of endoscopy. It is as accurate as conventional endoscopy in detecting abnormalities of the esoph-

The PillCam ESO is a safe, noninvasive, convenient, and patient-friendly test that could revolutionize screening in GERD. Screening is extremely important, as 10 to 15 percent of patients with chronic GERD symptoms will have Barrett's esophagus, a pre-cancerous condition that may lead to esophageal cancer.

~

Forty-eight-hour pH monitoring tells how long and how often the pH of the esophagus is acidic. This is the gold standard test for diagnosing GERD.

agus such as Barrett's. (Note, however, that if patients have symptoms consistent with other problems in the GI tract, such as ulcers, the PillCam may not detect problems in the stomach or the small intestines.)

The Bravo pH Monitoring System

EGD (endoscopy) and PillCam ESO are used to visualize the lining of the esophagus. This easily identifies patients with erosive esophagitis, Barrett's esophagus, and esophageal cancer. However, since a majority of patients with GERD have the non-erosive type, NERD, the doctor may not be able to see damage in the esophagus with either an endoscopy or a PillCam. In this case, another option for diagnosing GERD is to check how much and how often acid comes up into the esophagus. This is done by pH monitoring.

Before the Bravo pH Monitoring System was introduced in 2003 by Medtronic, the only way to measure pH levels in the esophagus was to place a catheter down the nose into the esophagus. The patient was required to leave the catheter in for twenty-four hours, which caused nasal discomfort and embarrassment about being seen with the catheter.

Bravo is the world's only catheter-free pH monitoring system, making it a very patient-friendly procedure. The test involves

Open Up and Say, "Ah!"

implantation of a miniature pH capsule in the esophagus during endoscopy. The capsule transmits pH readings to an external receiver, which the patient wears on his or her belt. The patient documents in a diary all the symptoms that occur during the next forty-eight hours. The capsule eventually sloughs off and passes in the stool. Some patients may feel a vague "foreign body sensation" in their esophagus; this, of course, is temporary. (Note that patients with pacemakers or implantable defibrillators cannot use Bravo.) After forty-eight hours, the data is uploaded into a computer, where it is then interpreted by the physician. On reviewing the Bravo results, the physician will be able to tell the number of refluxes the patient had, the duration of the refluxes, the number of refluxes longer than five minutes, and the time pH was less than four, correlating these findings with the patient's symptom diary. This test generates an overall score, called the Johnson DeMeester Score, which helps the physician determine the presence and severity of GERD.

More and more this test is being

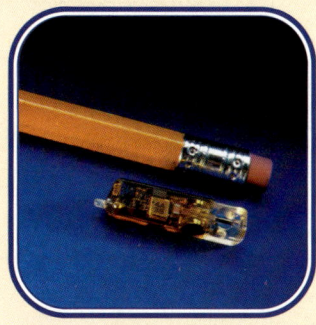

FIGURE 22A
Bravo capsule size compared to a standard pencil.

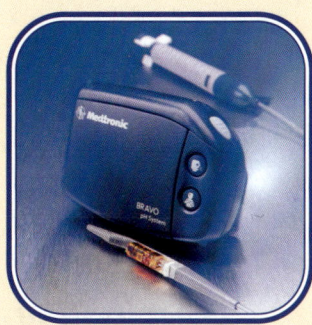

FIGURE 22B
Bravo Receiver with pH capsule and delivery system.

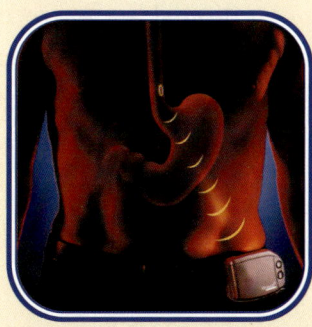

FIGURE 22C
Bravo pH capsule in use.

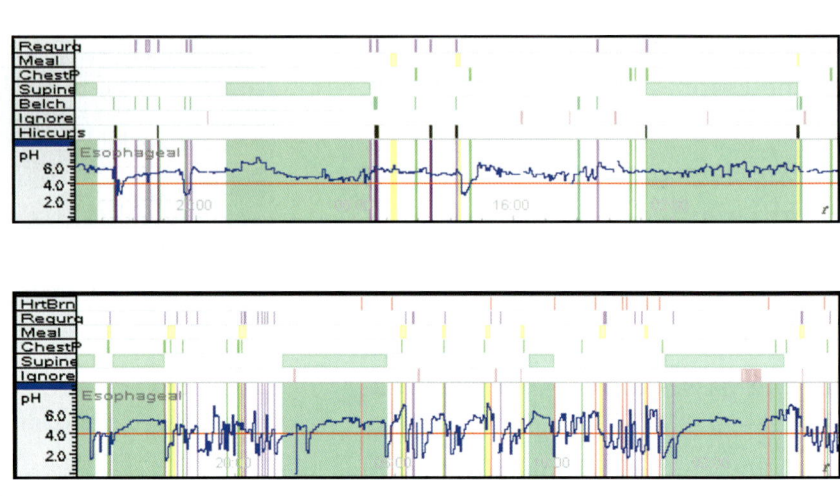

FIGURE 23A & 23B: Top is a normal reading. Bottom figure shows a patient with GERD.

used to diagnose reflux in patients with NERD, especially if they have atypical symptoms, and also to document the severity of the disease in patients who are getting ready for surgery.

Other Testing Methods

There are several other tests that have been used in the past and still are occasionally used to diagnose GERD. It has been shown, however, that these tests are not as accurate as the tests mentioned in the preceding sections. These tests include the barium esophagram/upper gastrointestinal series, esophageal motility study, impedance testing, and provocative testing.

The barium esophagram/upper gastrointestinal series (GI series) is rarely used today to diagnose GERD. Although it is less expensive, it is not a good test to diagnose GERD. It is a good test

Open Up and Say, "Ah!"

REFLUX TABLE — Acid Reflux Analysis & Total

FACTOR	TOTAL	UPRIGHT	SUPINE
Duration of Period (HH:MM)	1d, 20:05	1d, 01:22	18:42
Number of Refluxes	150	136	17
Number of Long Refluxes (>5 (min))	29	26	5
Duration of longest reflux (min)	42	29	33
Time pH < 4 ((min))	420	332	88
Fraction time pH < 4 ((%))	15	21.8	7.9

Johnson-DeMeester Score — Total
Total score = 73.4, Johnson-DeMeester (normal = less than 22 (95th percentile)

SAP TABLE — Total

FACTOR	TOTAL	SORE THROAT	HICCUPS
HrtBrn	88.2	0.0	0.0
Regurg	100.0	0.0	0.0
ChestP	86.2	0.0	0.0
Belch	0.0	0.0	0.0

SI TABLE — Total

FACTOR	TOTAL	SORE THROAT	HICCUPS
HrtBrn	20	n/a	n/a
Regurg	38.1	n/a	n/a
ChestP	18.2	n/a	n/a
Belch	n/a	n/a	n/a

FIGURE 23C: Bravo readings of patient with severe GERD

for the diagnosis of hiatal hernia, but as mentioned previously, you can have a hiatal hernia and not have GERD, and vice versa.

The esophageal motility study is also not a good test for diagnosing GERD. If you are diagnosed with GERD and are being considered for surgery, this test is done to be sure that the esophagus is working right. This is important for surgical patients, because if the esophagus is not functioning correctly due to

> If you are taking any medications for GERD, check with your physician about whether to stop taking those medications before a Bravo pH test. This decision will vary on a case by case determination.
>
> ~
>
> *I had two endoscopies and was told my esophagus looked normal. The implication was that my acid reflux was all in my head. But I continued to have symptoms, and in frustration, I went to another doctor. He ordered a Bravo test and said after seeing the results that I was the worst case of acid reflux he had ever seen. I guess I have NERD, the non-erosive type of reflux.*
> —Teresa, age 63

inadequate or uncoordinated peristalsis, the condition may actually be worsened by "tightening" the sphincter. The esophageal motility study involves placing a catheter into the stomach via the nose and checking the pressure of the esophagus and the lower esophageal sphincter. The patient is awake for this procedure, so it is uncomfortable.

Impedance testing and provocative testing are two other tests that are rarely used for GERD diagnosis and are only available at very specialized centers.

It doesn't take a genius to diagnose GERD. Most physicians make a clinical diagnosis based on the patient's description of symptoms. But the tests described in this chapter may be essential to determine that there are no complications — especially esophageal cancer — to the disease. Fortunately, technological strides forward in the past few years in diagnostic capabilities are aiding this diagnostic process.

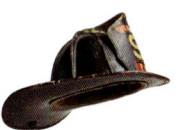

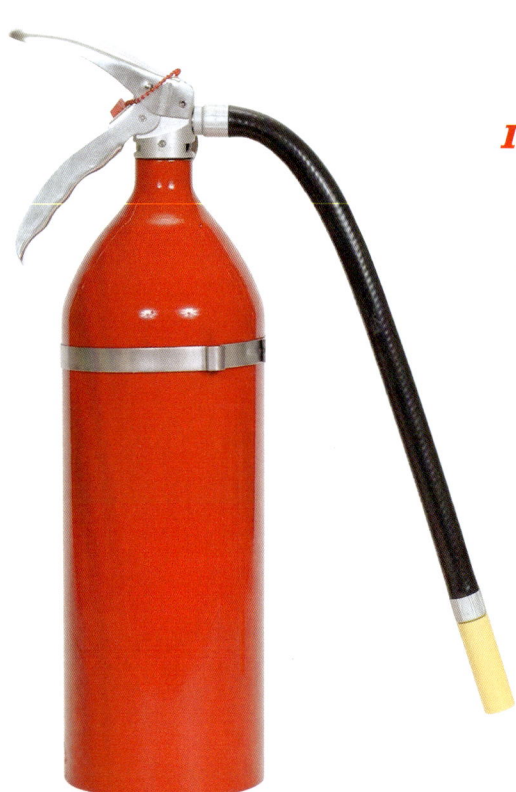

In this chapter...
- Lifestyle changes to treat GERD
- Medical or pharmacological treatment of GERD
- Endoscopic and surgical treatment of GERD

Chapter Six
Pills, Knife, or No More Spice

Pain is inevitable. Suffering is optional.
~ Anonymous

Treatment Options for GERD

Americans suffering from heartburn and other GERD symptoms spend more than two billion dollars on over-the-counter medications each year. That's in addition to the ten billion dollars spent annually on prescription medications to fight this disease.

The trend of treating reflux disease with over-the-counter medications has increased because in recent years the FDA approved the sale of all classes of GERD medications without a prescription, particularly the PPIs (proton pump inhibitors such as Prilosec).

But despite the temptation to treat GERD without the advice and assistance of a physician, it is always best that medical conditions like this be monitored by a professional.

There are five basic goals of GERD treatment:
- Resolve symptoms and make the patient feel better (This is the primary goal.)
- Heal inflammation (esophagitis), if present
- Prevent complications
- Improve quality of life
- Maintain remission

Remember, GERD is a chronic condition, just like high blood pressure or diabetes. Treatment usually is long-term, and without maintenance therapy, most patients with the erosive esophagitis type of GERD will find that symptoms reoccur within three months. For those with NERD, 75 percent of patients relapse within six months.

For those suffering from mild GERD, it's often easy to get by with "on demand" therapy — meaning people treat themselves on an as-needed basis. If you are still having symptoms in spite of strong medications, you should always consult a physician, as the initial diagnosis may have been wrong. Your physician can help you decide about further testing or other medications to try.

There are several ways to treat GERD, all of which are effective depending on the patient's situation and degree of disease: lifestyle change, medical treatment (a challenge because the stomach produces two liters of acid *every* day), endoscopic treatment, and surgical treatment.

Lifestyle Changes

For the majority of GERD patients, lifestyle modifications alone rarely solve their problems. But there are things that people can

Pills, Knife, or No More Spice

do to minimize their symptoms and improve quality of life, such as avoiding large meals and bedtime snacks and using common sense in food choices. If certain foods cause worsening of symptoms, stop eating them. But if you must eat those foods, take medication in anticipation of the meal (a histamine$_2$ blocker or a fast-acting PPI).

Here are some other things to consider.

- Avoid peppermint, chocolate, and fatty foods, as they are known to increase reflux by decreasing the lower esophageal sphincter pressure.

- Avoid refluxogenic foods such as coffee, citrus juices, spicy foods, tomatoes, colas and carbonated beverages. Individual patients may find that different foods cause their GERD symptoms to worsen. (Note: Tea usually does not cause reflux.)

- Avoid lying down right after eating. It varies for individuals, but for most people, it works to avoid eating for two hours before bedtime.

- Lie on your left side while sleeping, rather than your right side.

- Eat a low-fat and high-protein diet.

- Elevate the head of your bed using a six-inch block. Don't just pile up the pillows, as that will only elevate your head and you need to raise the upper torso, too. A foam wedge

> Visit www.spurntheburn.com for information on special pillows that help decrease nocturnal reflux.
>
> ~
>
> *I began treating myself with antacids, and they worked for a while. Then I kept gaining weight, so I had to go to a doctor for stronger medication. I went on Zantac, but even now, it doesn't work all the time, and I sometimes need additional medicine.*
>
> ~ Carrie, age 50

to raise the upper body may help as well.

- Lose weight if you're overweight. Obesity tends to exacerbate GERD.

- Stop smoking and avoid excessive alcohol use.

- Examine the medications you are taking to determine if any of them exacerbate reflux. (See the list of medications that may cause trouble in chapter 2, "Burn, Baby, Burn!")

- Avoid wearing tight clothes.

Despite all these precautions, most patients will need some type of medication. For some, the idea of giving up much-loved foods or changing other lifestyle habits is stressful and affects quality of life negatively. Keep in mind that it is fine to indulge occasionally if GERD symptoms resolve upon medical treatment.

Pharmacological Management or Medical Management?

There are two primary ways that medical professionals tackle GERD. The first is to decrease or stop the primary problem — in other words, trying to keep the acid inside the stomach. That means stopping the reflux of acid into the esophagus, which can

Pills, Knife, or No More Spice

be done with some medications (called promotility agents) or through surgical or endoscopic procedures. The second way is to decrease the gastric volume and acidity. This can be done with medications called H_2 blockers or PPIs (proton pump inhibitors).

Antacids

Antacids rarely help as the only treatment for GERD. They do help with immediate relief of symptoms, but because the duration of action is short, frequent dosing is necessary. They also do not heal the esophagitis, making antacids a poor therapeutic choice for treating GERD patients.

Antacids are neutralizing compounds that include aluminum- or magnesium-based calcium carbonate, magnesium, and/or sodium bicarbonate. Commonly, they are used as an adjunctive therapy to H_2 blockers or PPIs. For patients on those medications who have breakthrough symptoms (symptoms that occur while taking medicine on a regular basis), antacids can help alleviate the problem.

Taking antacids can have side effects. Calcium-based antacids can increase calcium in the bloodstream and in some instances, can actually increase acid production. Aluminum-based antacids

---

The goal of medical treatment is to bring the pH above 4.0 for as long a period as possible. Antacids and Carafate help by temporarily neutralizing the acid.

~

Acid, along with other enzymes in the stomach, breaks down food into smaller pieces. Suppression of acid with medications does not seem to negatively affect the process of digestion.

~

Antacids work locally and are not absorbed. They are, therefore, safe for pregnant women.

can cause constipation and magnesium-based products can cause diarrhea.

Gaviscon is the only antacid approved by the FDA in the treatment of GERD. In addition to aluminum and magnesium, Gaviscon has alginic acid, which works as an anti-reflux agent by floating on top of the stomach acid, decreasing acid that refluxes into the esophagus. Although it is clear that Gaviscon helps with symptoms, it is less certain whether it actually heals inflammation.

Promotility Drugs or Prokinetic Drugs

As the name implies, promotility drugs work by increasing motility. Motility agents help by clearing the acid from the esophagus quickly and decreasing "contact time" — the amount of time that the acid is in contact with the lining of the esophagus. The only FDA-approved drug in this category is metoclopramide (Reglan). This works by increasing esophageal peristalsis and also by increasing lower esophageal sphincter pressure. It also speeds up the emptying of the stomach, which helps indirectly.

Unfortunately, there are numerous side effects, and patients should be careful when taking this medication. Possible side effects are drowsiness, headache, fatigue, lethargy, anxiety, depression, and Parkinson's symptoms that include tremors, rigidity, and tardive dyskinesia (a problem characterized by repetitive, involuntary, and purposeless movements).

Another drug occasionally used in this category is called bethanecol, which increases lower esophageal pressure. The following drugs are not approved for GERD but occasionally are pre-

Pills, Knife, or No More Spice

scribed: cisapride (brand name Propulsid), Domperidone, Zelnorm, Baclofen, and Erythromycin.

Acid Suppression Therapy — H_2RAs and PPIs

To understand how acid suppression therapy drugs work, it is important to discuss the secretion of stomach acid on a cellular level. Special cells, called parietal cells, in the stomach secrete hydrochloric acid. There are three types of receptors on these parietal cells: histamine$_2$, acetylcholine, and gastrin. Activation of these receptors stimulates the parietal cells, which in turn activates the proton pump, which then secretes the acid. Essentially, the proton pump (also called the gastric acid pump or the hydrogen potassium adenosine triphosphate pump) is the final pathway for gastric acid production.

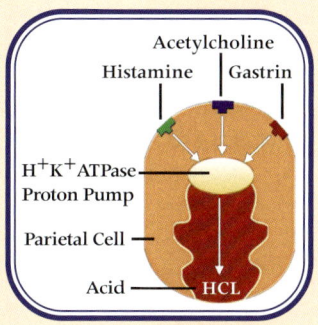

FIGURE 24A
Proton pump

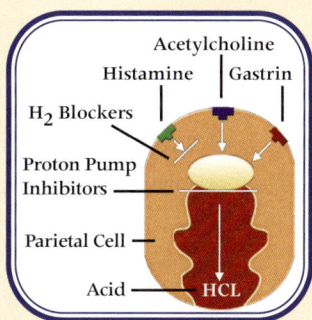

FIGURE 24B
Mechanism of action of drugs

H_2RAs and PPIs decrease the volume and the acidity (which means they increase the pH) of the acid that is secreted by the parietal cells. Doses of individual H_2RAs and PPIs vary depending on the individual medication used and upon the severity of the reflux. A physician will be able to determine the correct medication and dosage.

> The thought, sight, smell, and taste of food starts acid production in the stomach. This is because the brain is telling the stomach that it needs to get ready because food is on the way. Once food hits the stomach, acid production increases and the digestive process can last about four hours.

H_2RAs work by suppressing gastric acid production by blocking the H_2 receptors on the parietal cells. These drugs include cimetidine (Tagamet), ranitidine (Zantac), famotidine (Pepcid), and nizatidine (Axid). H_2RAs are approved for mild GERD; higher doses are used to treat severe GERD.

H_2RAs tend to work better for nighttime acid suppression. They often are not strong enough for patients with atypical symptoms and are less suitable for long-term use because patients may develop tachyphylaxis, or rapid development of immunity to the effects of a drug. These are, however, safe drugs, and their side effects are minimal and rare. Side effects could include nonspecific symptoms like headache, nausea, and diarrhea. With Tagamet (cimetidine), some patients experience gynecomastia, or enlargement of the breasts, and occasional impotence.

Proton pump inhibitors, or PPIs, currently are used as first-line therapy for GERD. They are "stronger" and more effective than H_2RAs as they work directly on the proton pump, stopping acid production that is activated by any of the pathways, unlike the H_2RAs. They definitely are superior to H_2RAs regarding symptom relief and healing of erosive esophagitis.

Omeprazole (Prilosec), approved by the FDA in 1989, revolutionized treatment of GERD. Since then, several other PPIs have come on the market, and more are in the making. Prilosec OTC became available over the counter in 2003 and is also available in generic form. Other PPIs include esomeprazole (Nexium), lan-

Pills, Knife, or No More Spice

soprazole (Prevacid), pantaprozole (Protonix), and rabeprazole (Aciphex).

Prilosec, Prevacid, and Nexium are available as capsules; for people who have difficulty swallowing, the capsules can be opened and the granules sprinkled on food products or in juices. Prevacid and Protonix are available in intravenous form if needed (e.g., in the case of hospitalized patients who cannot take oral medications). Prevacid is available in a suspension liquid and also in an orally disintegrating tablet. The new PPI kid on the block offered as a suspension liquid is Zegerid, which is essentially a rapid-acting omeprazole (like Prilosec) that may make sense if an on-demand PPI is needed. PPIs need to be taken fifteen to thirty minutes before meals, as the pump needs to be activated for them to work, and eating stimulates acid production. PPIs are only effective when there is sufficient acid in the stomach.

Side effects for PPIs usually are minor and may include headache, nausea, abdominal pain, and diarrhea. Time and again, concerns have been raised as to the long-term safety of PPIs based on studies with

If the patient has no response with a particular PPI, the physician may switch the patient to another PPI. There is a good chance the second medication will work.

~

If you are on a PPI and have nighttime acid reflux (called a breakthrough symptom), it is usually acceptable to add an H_2 blocker at night to take care of the problem. However, this should be done only on an as-needed basis, to decrease the possibility of becoming tolerant to the H_2 blocker.

~

If you are on a PPI and are not responding to treatment, it is possible that there is not adequate acid suppression. Consult your physician about increasing the dose or the possibility of endoscopic treatments or surgery. Remember that it is possible that the diagnosis was wrong in the first place.

> Talk with your physician regarding any interaction that could occur between medications you take in addition to a PPI.
>
> ~
>
> Pregnant and lactating women should not take PPIs unless absolutely necessary. All PPIs do cross the placental barrier and some of them are secreted into breast milk.

animal models at much higher doses. But these medications have been shown to have a safe record in humans.

Remember that PPIs are metabolized in the liver, so any other medication metabolized in the liver can cause a "drug-to-drug interaction," meaning that the time taken to clear the drug may be prolonged. Drug-to-drug interactions with PPIs vary from medication to medication. These may include but are not limited to the following drugs: Coumadin, Valium, Digoxin, and Biaxin. Check with your physician to determine if any drug you are taking could interact negatively with the PPI you are taking.

Other Medications

Carafate (sucralfate) is another drug used occasionally for the treatment of GERD. Data is limited as to its effectiveness in treating this disease, however, so it is not used commonly. It is an aluminum hydroxide salt of sucrose called octasulphate. It should be used with caution in patients with kidney problems and renal failure, as aluminum can cause dementia.

Sucralfate works by coating the esophagus, forming a protective layer to keep acid from getting into the esophagus. Like the antacids, sucralfate is not absorbed and can safely be used by pregnant women.

Pills, Knife, or No More Spice

Endoscopic Management

Endoscopic management means that a gastroenterologist repairs the sphincter through a scope. Gastroenterologists perform the procedure from inside the esophagus, unlike surgeries that are performed by a surgeon working from outside the body. There are various types of procedures done endoscopically, and each involves working on the lower esophageal sphincter: cooking (the Stretta procedure), stuffing (injection with Enteryx), sewing (endocinch procedure), the NDO plicator procedure, and the Gatekeeper.

Cooking, or the Stretta procedure, involves radio frequency "cooking" of the LES and the upper stomach. When the area heals, scar tissue is formed, which causes the tissue to contract as it heals. This helps in about 70 percent of patients (at least on a short-term basis). This procedure is not recommended if the patient has a hiatal hernia or Barrett's esophagus.

Stuffing, or injection with Enteryx, involves injecting the LES with a copolymer that serves to form a permanent implant in the LES, enhancing its efficiency.

Endocinch involves tightening the GE junction area, creating an artificial sphincter by putting sutures across the upper part of the stomach. The short-term success rate with this procedure is between 50 and 60 percent. There is not adequate data to determine long-term success rates. If the patient has a large hiatal hernia, this procedure cannot be done.

Another procedure, called the NDO plicator, was approved by the FDA in late 2004. As insurance companies are not reimbursing for this procedure, very few centers are doing it. The NDO plicator involves a specialist putting a full thickness plication

In preliminary studies, it appears the Gatekeeper is safe, effective, and reversible, and significantly improves symptoms and quality of life in patients with GERD.

~

Endoscopic management for GERD is still in its infancy and there is little data on long-term results. Moreover, it is done by only a few gastroenterologists in specialized centers throughout the country. Visit with your physician about whether you are a candidate for endoscopic treatment.

(stitch), using an endoscope, at the gastroesophageal junction. Preliminary one-year results for this endoscopic option look good, but no long-term data is available.

Recently approved for use in Europe is a new endoscopic anti-reflux technique, the Gatekeeper reflux repair system. It has not yet been approved by the FDA and is not commercially available in the United States. This new, *reversible* treatment modality involves endoscopic introduction of a prosthesis into the esophageal submucosa to augment the lower esophageal sphincter.

The prosthesis is made of expandable polyacrylonitrile-based hydrogel. Preliminary results are promising. Studies have shown that in a significant number of patients, LES pressure increases significantly and symptoms decrease dramatically with this procedure.

Surgical Management

Although most GERD patients can be managed by lifestyle changes and medication, there is a small group of patients that will benefit from surgery. In most cases, surgery can be done laparoscopically (through several small incisions), and the recovery time is relatively minimal.

Patients who may benefit from surgery include those who have been unable to control symptoms with medical treatment

Pills, Knife, or No More Spice

or those whose symptoms are controlled but prefer surgery over taking medicines on a long-term basis. This subset would include young patients (less than fifty years) as they may not want to take medicines for thirty years or more, because the average life span of Americans is exceeding eighty years nowadays.

After the decision has been made to proceed with surgery, several tests must be performed. An EGD (esophagogastroduodenoscopy) and a forty-eight-hour pH study with Bravo must be done to document the diagnosis and severity of reflux. Sometimes these procedures already will have been done as part of the diagnostic process. If the patient has had an EGD and erosive esophagitis was diagnosed, the physician or surgeon may decide not to do this test.

An esophageal motility study is performed to make sure the esophagus is working properly. For this test, a catheter is placed through the nose in the esophagus and the stomach and the patient is asked to swallow water. Esophageal pressures are recorded to make sure that the peristalsis process is working correctly. If there is a problem with peristalsis, the surgeon may adapt the surgical procedure to accommodate for what is called a "failed esophagus," or an esophagus that doesn't work properly. Usually, the surgeon will decide to do a partial wrap (toupet procedure) instead of a full wrap (See an example of this in Figures 25a-25d.).

The surgery, which takes about an hour, is called Nissen fundoplication and involves "wrapping" the upper portion of the stomach (the fundus) around the lower esophagus. If the patient has a hiatal hernia, this is "reduced" during the procedure, and the surgeon sutures the hiatal opening to make it

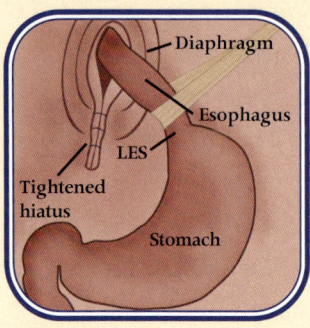

FIGURE 25A
Tightened hiatus

~

I tried every medicine available to treat my GERD. Nothing worked and I continued to have many symptoms. The surgery worked well; I am much improved. The only side effect has been that I can't belch.

~ Damon, age 65

~

When choosing a surgeon to perform laparoscopic anti-reflux surgery, it is important to make sure he or she has performed at least twenty-five of these surgeries. Experience is an important factor in the success of this surgery.

"tight." Surgery typically is performed laparoscopically through several small incisions on the abdomen. Occasionally an "open" surgery may be necessary; the chance of this happening is higher if the patient has had previous upper abdominal surgery because adhesions may make the laparoscopic procedure difficult. The success rate of surgery with an experienced surgeon could be as high as 80 or 90 percent.

Risks and Side Effects of Surgery

Infection and bleeding are risks in every surgery, but the incidence is low after laparoscopic surgery. There is a very small risk of perforation of either the esophagus or the stomach during surgery. If this should happen, the surgeon may have to switch from a laparoscopic surgery to an open procedure.

Dysphagia (difficulty swallowing) occurs for a short time in all patients. This will usually resolve in four to six weeks, but if it persists (and this sometimes happens) the patient may need esophageal dilatation, a technique that

Pills, Knife, or No More Spice

opens the blocked portion of the esophagus.

Some patients may experience "gas bloat syndrome," which occurs when air gets trapped in the stomach. This usually resolves in a few months. The inability to belch also happens occasionally and can cause nausea.

There is a slight risk of injury to bowel or blood vessels with placement of trocars, a surgical instrument needed for all laparoscopic surgeries.

The vast majority of GERD patients can be treated successfully with medication therapy. For those who need additional treatment, there is much research being done. As surgical and endoscopic options continue to improve and advance, it is hoped that physicians will be able to improve the quality of life successfully for most patients suffering from this disease.

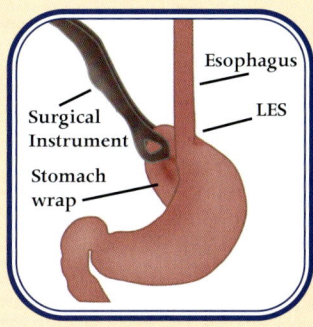

FIGURE 25B
The stomach being wrapped around the esophagus

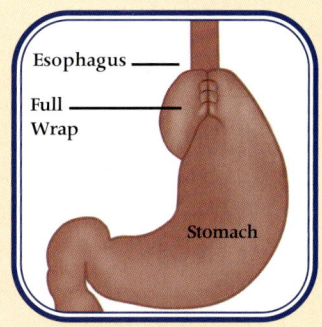

FIGURE 25C
A full wrap goes all the way around the LES (360° wrap)

Treatment Options for the Complications of GERD

The treatment options for esophageal stricture, Barrett's esophagus, as well as esophageal cancer are discussed briefly in chapter 4, "What Went Wrong?" However, the treatment of these serious health issues can be multi-faceted and complex. Please consult your doctor for more information regarding treatment options for these conditions.

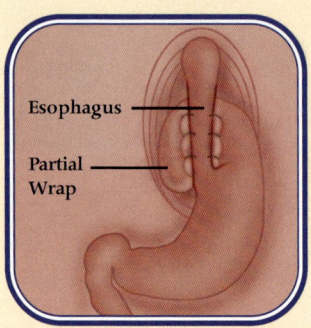

FIGURE 25D
A partial wrap does not go all the way around the esophagus

~

See chapter 4, "What Went Wrong?" for more information about treatment options for esophageal stricture, Barrett's esophagus, and esophageal cancer.

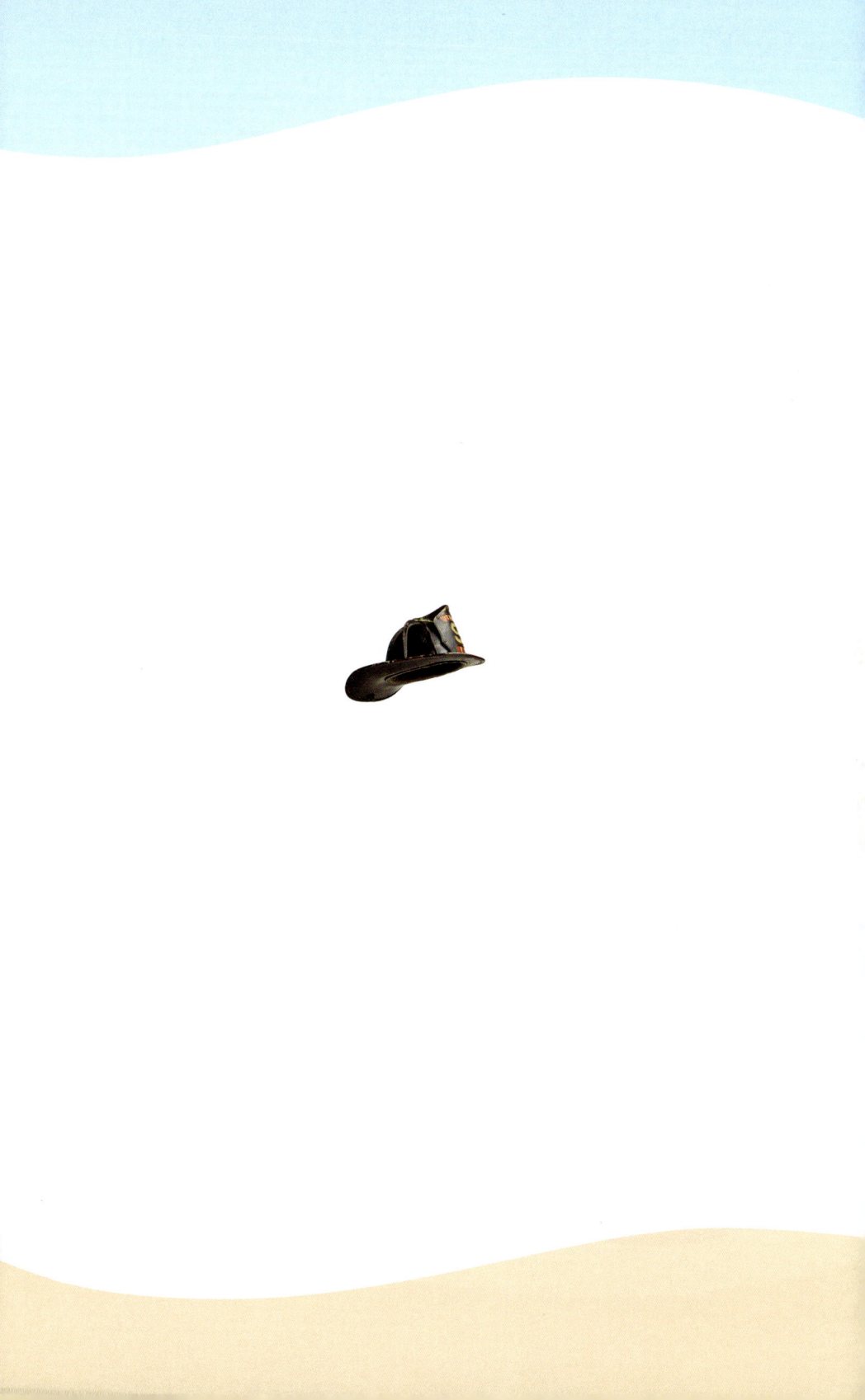

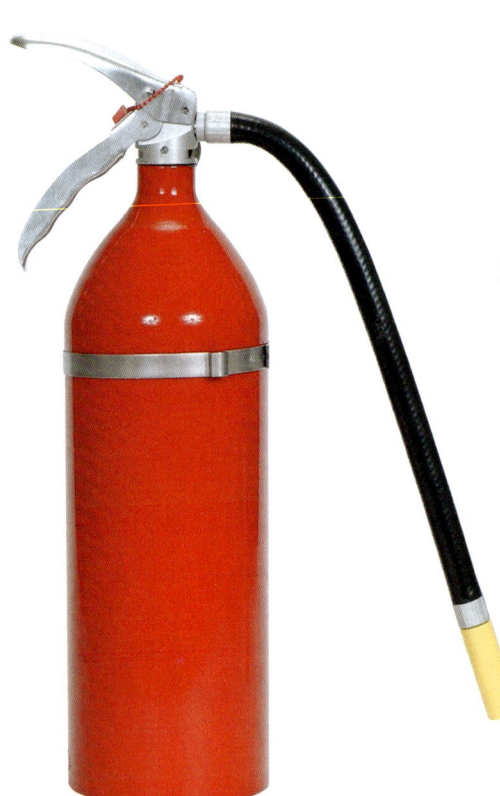

In this chapter...

- Alternative treatment for GERD
- Carminative herbs
- Bitter digestive stimulants

Chapter Seven
A Spot of Chamomile Tea

Following the Romanian tradition, garlic is used in excess to keep the vampires away. Following the Jewish tradition, a dispenser of schmaltz (liquid chicken fat) is kept on the table to give the vampires heartburn if they get through the garlic defense.
~ Calvin Trillin

Herbal and Alternative Treatments for GERD

An interest in alternative and complementary medicine — which includes everything from megavitamin therapy to acupuncture to prayer — has been increasing in the United States for many years.

Healthcare spending patterns have followed that interest. The most recent spending research was National Health Interview Survey and dates from 1997. At that time, Americans spent an estimated $36 billion to $47 billion on alternative and complementary medicine. Of this amount, about $5 billion was for out-of-pocket spending on herbal products.

Spurn the Burn

> Author's Note: As a traditional doctor, I have little experience with or knowledge about herbs and alternative medical treatments. But based on reader feedback from my other book, *Winning the Hepatitis C Battle*, I have chosen to include this chapter. I would urge anyone using or considering herbal remedies to talk with their physician.

If you choose to treat GERD with any alternative medicines, be sure to keep your physician informed. Herbal medicines can interact with prescriptions in some cases and also may have side effects of which you are unaware.

Literature on herbal remedies for GERD is abundant and often contradictory. There are literally dozens of herbal remedies for heartburn and few that are specifically touted as cures or treatment for GERD. As with the majority of herbal medicines, devotees claim that most have minimal side effects.

Unlike traditional drugs, the FDA does not regulate herbal remedies and treatments, and therefore, their true effectiveness is often difficult to judge. Moreover, a prepackaged treatment for heartburn often contains many different herbs, some of which are not combating heartburn itself. A variety of sources however, including the American Botanical Council, advocate the use of chamomile (Matricaria recutita) and ginger (Zingiber officinale) to treat this condition.

Chamomile, widely recognized for its calming properties, is thought to help relieve esophageal irritation and aid proper digestion. It is presumed to work through decreasing stomach acid, due to its high calcium content. Traditionally used for many gastrointestinal problems, ginger assists in proper digestion by promoting spontaneous intestinal movement. In addition, ginger has anti-inflammatory and anti-nausea properties. Those who are allergic to ragweed or other plants in the Aster-

A Spot of Chamomile Tea

aceae family (including echinacea, feverfew and chrysanthemums) should avoid chamomile.

These herbs fall into a group of herbs the General Nutrition Center (GNC) terms "carminative" (medicines thought to relieve gas in the alimentary tract or ease its passing) and are believed to relieve indigestion and intestinal irritation. Among the most notable and well-studied carminatives are fennel, caraway, and wormwood. These have been found to reduce gas, cramping, and indigestion.

> Although heartburn can often be alleviated with antacids and other modern medicines, some patients prefer to pursue relief via herbal remedies. The most commonly cited herbal remedies for heartburn are chamomile, ginger, aloe vera, and licorice.

In addition to the carminative class of heartburn herbs, GNC also suggests that "bitter digestive stimulants" such as blessed thistle may promote digestive enzyme production and alleviate heartburn. However, such herbs are not as universally recommended as chamomile, ginger, and peppermint.

To follow is a summary of treatments frequently recommended by those practicing alternative medicine:

- **Licorice root, meadowsweet, chamomile, and lemon** are some herbs believed to treat heartburn and decrease stomach acid. Also consider herbs that absorb excess acid: slippery elm, marshmallow, flax, and fenugreek seeds. Since the malic and tartaric acids in carrots and apples also neutralize stomach acid, consider combining the juices of these vegetables with the herbs to make an extra-tasty tea. "Clinical studies" (there is some controversy over how scientific these studies are) have shown that chamomile, marshmallow,

> Caution: The use of herbs is a time-honored approach to strengthening the body and treating disease. Herbs, however, contain active substances that can trigger side effects and interact with other herbs, supplements, or medications. For these reasons, herbs should be taken with care, under the supervision of a practitioner knowledgeable in the field of botanical medicine.

licorice, slippery elm, calendula, garlic, wild yam, and St. John's wort protect the stomach from its own acid and also reduce inflammation and infection of the lining.

- **Catnip** can potentially aid in promoting proper digestion.

- **Ginger** is another potential digestion aid. This herbal remedy is most popular for its usefulness in battling motion sickness and reducing nausea.

- **Licorice (Glycyrrhiza glabra)** is a flavorful herb that has been used in food and medicinal remedies for thousands of years. This herb has long been valued as a demulcent (soothing, coating agent) and continues to be used by professional herbalists today to relieve respiratory ailments (e.g., allergies, bronchitis, colds, sore throats, tuberculosis), stomach problems (including, possibly, heartburn from reflux or some other cause and gastritis), inflammatory disorders, skin diseases, and liver problems. High doses of licorice (more than twenty grams per day) may cause serious side effects. It is important to consult a physician about how much to take. Problems can be avoided if doses are kept within recommended guidelines. People with high blood pressure, obesity, diabetes, or kidney, heart, or liver conditions should avoid licorice. Use of any licorice product is not recommended for longer than four to six weeks.

- **Marshmallow root, papaya, fennel, and catnip teas** may ease heartburn.

- **Turmeric (Curcuma longa)** is sometimes recommended for GERD symptoms. Turmeric has long been used in both Ayurvedic and Chinese medicine to treat digestive disorders. Scientific research is beginning to test the merit of this traditional use. In an animal study, for example, extracts of turmeric root reduced the release of acid from the stomach and protected against injuries such as inflammation and ulcers, both of which are potential complications from GERD. (Note: At very high doses, turmeric may induce ulcers. It is very important to stick with the dose recommended by an herbal specialist.) People who have gallstones should not take turmeric.

- **Aloe vera juice** aids healing of the intestinal tract and has been used for ages in treating "agitated esophagus." The plant extract contains naturally occurring pectin, which is supposed to help GERD.

- **Dill** soothes the digestive tract. Crushed seeds are best. They can be used in a salad dressing or in other recipes for cooking. Caution: Those who are pregnant should use dill in moderation.

- **Centaurium** is recommended for indigestion, heartburn, and acid reflux. This product is not recommended for women who are pregnant or nursing unless directed by a health care professional.

- **Stomach bitters** are generally used to improve digestion. They do so by increasing the secretion of digestive enzymes, increasing gut motility, and tighten the esophageal sphincter. Tightening the esophageal sphincter reduces the tendency for reflux of the gastric contents into the esophagus, a condition that is seen with hiatal hernia and other causes of reflux and gives rise to the symptom of heartburn.

- **Nux vomica** is recommended for heartburn, nausea, retching without vomiting, and sour burps caused by overeating, alcohol use, or coffee drinking; this remedy is most appropriate for individuals who also feel irritable and sensitive to noise and light.

- **Relief chi** is a natural Chinese herbal supplement used for heartburn relief. It contains a soothing plant enzyme that works on the part of the central nervous system that regulates digestion and aids in the breakdown of food for proper digestion and assimilation of nutrients.

- **Slippery elm** in powdered form, mixed with a little water, may be used for GERD symptoms. The mucilage content in slippery elm appears to act as a barrier against the damaging effects of acid on the esophagus in people with heartburn.

A Spot of Chamomile Tea

- **Artichoke,** in addition to being an edible plant, is a mild bitter. Extracts of artichoke have been repeatedly shown in double-blind research to be beneficial for people with indigestion.

- **Boldo** has been used in South America for a variety of digestive conditions. Studies specifically showing a benefit from taking boldo in people with indigestion and heartburn have not been performed.

- **Linden** has long been used for indigestion. Older clinical trials have shown that linden flower tea can help people who suffer from upset stomach or from excessive gas.

- **Numerous carminative herbs,** including European angelica root (Angelica archangelica), anise, basil, lemon balm, cardamom, cinnamon, cloves, coriander, dill, ginger, oregano, rosemary, sage, lavender, and thyme are common kitchen herbs and thus are readily available for making tea to calm an upset stomach. Rosemary is sometimes used to treat indigestion in the elderly by European herbal practitioners. Green tea has been used for centuries in Japan for helping with acid reflux and indigestion.

- **Fresh papaya or pineapple** may aid digestion. Chewing a few of the papaya seeds as well. Papaya enzyme chewable tablets can be a substitute for fresh papaya.

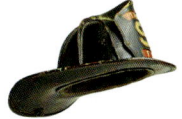

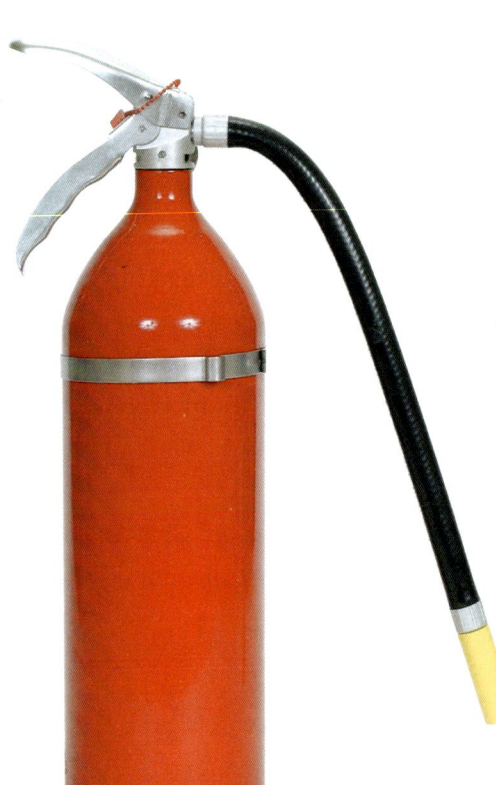

In this chapter...
- Helicobacter Pylori and GERD
- Pregnancy and GERD
- GERD in children and the elderly

Chapter Eight
Bugs, Mommies, Babies, and Grannies

Pain is not evil unless it conquers us.
~ George Eliot

Helicobacter Pylori and GERD

It is clear that infection from the bacteria Helicobacter pylori is a major factor in the development of inflammation and/or ulcers in the stomach and small intestines. It is felt that this bacterium is linked to some stomach cancers and lymphomas. An H.Pylori infection is often treated with PPIs and antibiotics.

The relationship between this bacteria and GERD is unclear. It is believed by some experts that H.Pylori is actually a protective mechanism in GERD. In contrast, other experts think there is no relationship between H.Pylori infection of the stomach and

Spurn the Burn

> Myth or fact? If you have heartburn during pregnancy, your baby will be born with a lot of hair. Go to www.spurn-theburn.com to find out.

GERD. Until the relationship is clearer, it is best for the gastroenterologist to treat H.Pylori if he or she feels it is causing the inflammation or ulceration in the stomach or duodenum.

Pregnancy and GERD

Heartburn in pregnancy is very common, sometimes quoted as occurring in as many as 75 percent of pregnant women. The incidence of GERD in pregnancy also is very high at more than 25 percent. Recurrence with subsequent pregnancies is very common, and symptoms tend to get worse as pregnancy advances.

The reason for this is twofold: The mechanical effect of the fetus pressing on the stomach can cause heartburn, and hormonal changes such as the increase in estrogens and progesterones during pregnancy causes the LES to relax, worsening GERD.

Also, some women wait too long before switching to maternity clothes, and tight clothes might contribute to the condition. Changing eating habits, such as ingestion of more refluxogenic foods, might contribute.

It is important to use care in treating GERD during pregnancy, as some medications may affect the fetus. Depending on the degree of risk, drugs are classified into different categories: A, B, C, D, and X. Drugs in categories A and B are considered safe. Be careful with using any drugs classified as C, D, or X.

All antacids are in category A, and all H_2 blockers are in category B (Tagamet, Zantac, Pepcid, and Axid). PPIs are probably

Bugs, Mommies, Babies, and Grannies

safe, but not enough research data is available. Most PPIs are in category B, with the exception of Prilosec, which is a category C drug.

GERD in Infants and Children

This is a brief summary regarding the difficulties of GERD in children. Please consult a pediatrician for specific information.

> *I was four months pregnant the first time I had heartburn. I checked with my doctor, and he said to take Tums. I did and it helped for a short time. Then my acid reflux got so bad that I would wake up at night, even vomiting a few times. Thank goodness the doctor could prescribe a safe medication to help me.*
>
> ~ Morgan, age 34

GERD is actually a common disease in infancy and may affect between 10 and 20 percent of infants. But the good news is that most babies outgrow their reflux by the time they are toddlers. Babies can be difficult to diagnose, but consider reflux disease if the baby cries a lot, stays up a lot, spits up a lot, or has recurrent vomiting. Hoarseness, persistent cough, recurrent hiccups, or persistent choking episodes may also be the signs of reflux in infants.

In older children, in addition to the reflux symptoms described in this book, look for worsening asthma at night, recurrent ear infections, recurrent vomiting, and weight loss due to refusal to eat.

If you or your pediatrician suspect reflux, it is best to be referred to a pediatric gastroenterologist who deals with reflux in children on a regular basis.

GERD and the Elderly

As the elderly population in the United States is growing, this is an important subgroup of GERD patients. It would appear that

> In elderly patients, the symptoms may be minimal, but GERD could be severe and complicated. Treatment should be aggressive and indefinite.

elderly patients may often have less severe symptoms, but paradoxically they have more severe disease than younger people. In addition, elderly individuals have a higher incidence of GERD complications. Therefore, treatment of the elderly suffering from GERD should be indefinite (lifelong).

Here are some reasons why elderly patients have more severe disease:

- Esophageal peristalsis decreases with advancing age; therefore, reflux episodes are longer.
- Hiatal hernias occur more frequently and are larger with advancing age.
- Elderly patients have decreased esophageal sensitivity to acid.
- They may be on multiple medications, some of which might relax the lower esophageal sphincter.
- Elderly patients are more inclined to lie down flat for longer periods of time, which is when they lose the advantage of gravity.

When examining the special situations around GERD, it is clear what a universal disease this is, including in its ranks everyone from child to the elderly. Heartburn can sometimes take a backseat to more "serious" illnesses and may not get the attention it deserves in elderly patients. For children, it often isn't considered as a possibility right away. But no matter who heartburn and

Bugs, Mommies, Babies, and Grannies

GERD affect, these conditions can severely affect quality of life and must be treated with the seriousness this disease deserves.

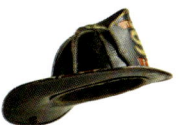

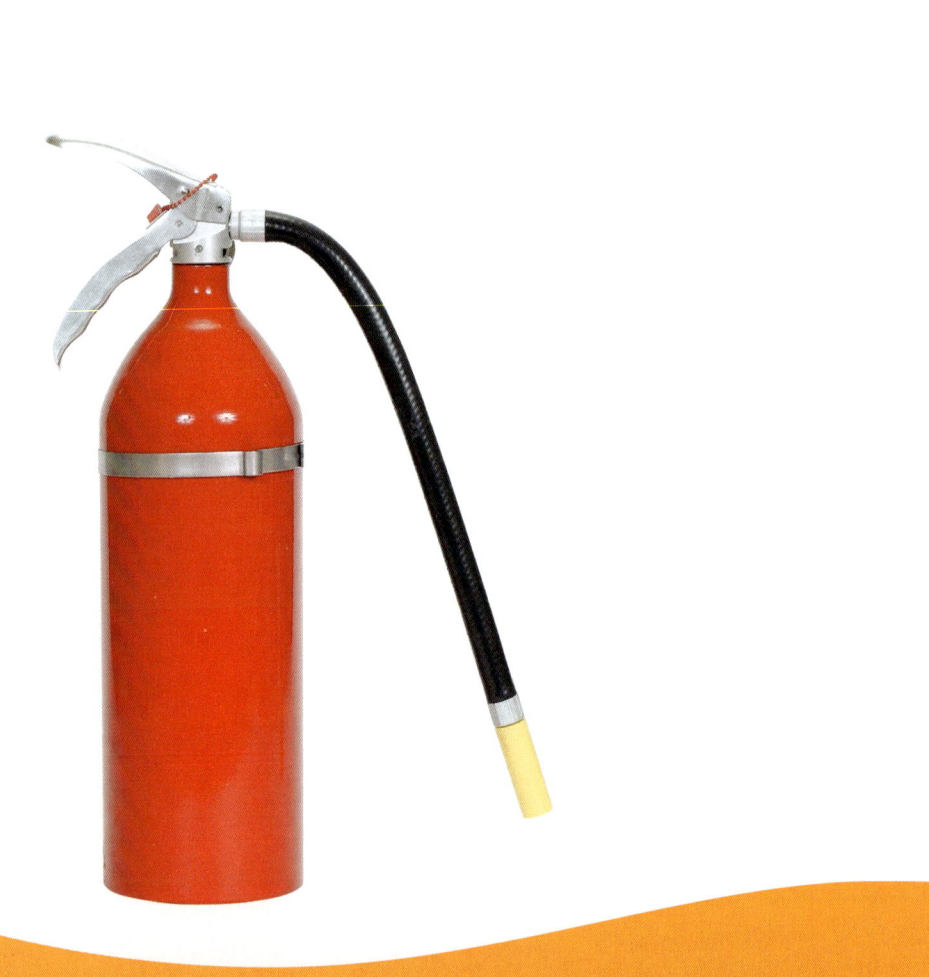

Afterword

After years of treating patients with GERD, I still am amazed at the wide disparity of symptoms and effects caused by this disease. There are patients who complain of mild symptoms that they treat with over-the-counter medications, whereas others lose sleep and suffer tremendous loss of quality of life.

The vast majority of the patients I see are treated easily with medication. Yet, GERD cannot be underestimated, because there is the group of people who suffer from the many complications of the disease. Most don't even know when they first walk in the doors of my practice that a simple thing like heartburn can be the harbinger of the pre-cancerous condition Barrett's esophagus or, even worse, esophageal cancer.

Thankfully, in the seventeen years of my practice, the medical profession has stepped up to help the sixty million people who suffer heartburn on a frequent basis. The effectiveness of medications has helped many people either completely eradicate their symptoms or control them sufficiently to feel little effects from GERD's symptoms. The introduction of PPIs, proton pump inhibitors, in the late 1980s remains the biggest stride forward for GERD medications.

Technology also has given professionals the tools needed to make diagnoses. The Bravo pH monitoring system, the PillCam, and other advances make the diagnostic process more accurate and comfortable for patients.

Treatment of GERD and its complications, in addition to the pharmaceutical advances, has both changed and remained the same. One of the most common surgeries, Nissen fundoplication, has been around since the very first GERD surgery (performed by Dr. Rudolph Nissen) in 1954. It has been adapted over the years to become more comfortable for patients because it is now performed laparoscopically. Yet there are many procedures now being used, some in just a few areas of the country such as endocinch, Stretta, Enteryx, photodynamic therapy, and submucosal resection. Some of these offer much promise for future GERD treatment. Other procedures on the horizon, like the Gatekeeper and the NDO plicator, may also advance the field.

I felt compelled to write this book because so many of my patients didn't understand why they were suffering from GERD, what its aggravating factors are, what treatment options are available, and what the complications can be to this disease. I'm hoping too, that it will reach some of the people who are not seeking medical help — those people who buy bottles of antacids and never discuss their heartburn with a physician. So

Afterword

many don't understand that a small percentage of people will develop problems that can threaten their life.

As in most medical conditions, the key is education, and I hope that *Spurn the Burn* does its part to help in that process.

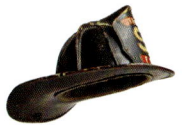

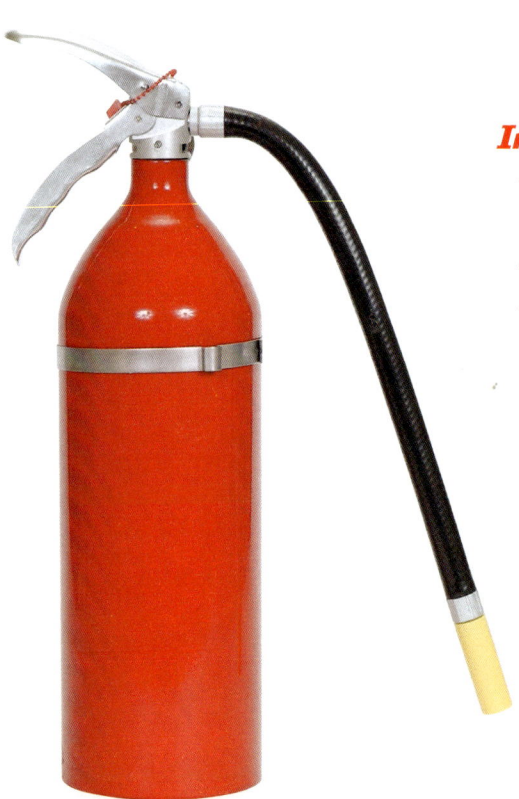

In this appendix...
- Symptoms and diagnosis of GERD
- Treatment of GERD
- Other questions you may have

Frequently Asked Questions

1. **What is GERD? Is it a common problem?**

    GERD, or gastroesophageal reflux disease, occurs when stomach acid backs up into the esophagus, causing damage to the esophagus and frequently disrupting quality of life. If symptoms (e.g., heartburn, acid reflux, chronic cough) occur two or more times a week, you should be checked for GERD.

    Yes, it is a very common problem.

2. **Is heartburn synonymous with GERD?**

    Heartburn is only one of the symptoms of GERD. If it occurs frequently, you may have GERD. However, you can have GERD without heartburn.

3. **What are some of the symptoms of GERD?**
   The classic symptom of GERD is heartburn. In addition, you may have regurgitation (effortless return of acidic stomach contents into the esophagus), waterbrash (excessive salivation), dysphagia (difficulty swallowing), odonophagia (painful swallowing), and upper abdominal pain. Atypical symptoms may include chest pain, chronic cough, asthma, repeated bronchial infections, hoarseness, dental decay, and so on.

4. **What causes GERD?**
   The lower esophageal sphincter, which is at the junction of the esophagus and the stomach, is a muscle that acts like a one-way valve (trap door) to prevent the acid from backing up into the esophagus. One cause of GERD is the failure of this sphincter to work correctly.

5. **Is there any difference between hiatal hernia and GERD?**
   Yes! A hiatal hernia occurs when part of the stomach comes into the chest through the diaphragmatic hiatus. One can have GERD and not have a hiatal hernia and vice versa.

6. **Can GERD be fatal? What are the problems I may face if I don't get checked?**
   Yes. GERD could be fatal. The complications of GERD include esophageal cancer (which is one of the deadliest cancers), esophageal stricture (narrowing of the esophagus), erosive esophagitis (inflammation of the esophagus) and Barrett's esophagus (a pre-cancerous condition).

Frequently Asked Questions

7. **What foods, medicines, and conditions exacerbate GERD?**
   Chocolate, caffeine, (coffee, tea, cola drinks), alcohol, peppermint, citrus juices, tomato products, spicy foods, raw onions, fatty foods, smoking, presence of a hiatal hernia, and gaining weight (obesity, pregnancy) all can exacerbate GERD. There are several medications that can exacerbate GERD; please refer to chapter 2, "Burn, Baby, Burn!" for a complete list. For additional recipes and diet advice, see Elaine Magee's book, *Tell Me What to Eat If I Have Acid Reflux*.

8. **Do most pregnant women get GERD? How can I handle GERD during my pregnancy?**
   GERD is very common during pregnancy. The mechanical effect of the fetus on the stomach and also the increase in hormones are responsible for this. Most of the antacids and H_2 blockers are safe to take during pregnancy. Please go to chapter 8, "Bugs, Mommies, Babies, and Grannies," to review what you can take while pregnant and also consult with your physician.

9. **How is GERD diagnosed?**
   For the most part, GERD is a clinical diagnosis, meaning if you have the classic symptoms, your physician will be able to diagnose GERD without any tests. The reason for testing is to make sure you do not have complicated GERD. The tests used to diagnose GERD or its complications include endoscopy, forty-eight-hour pH monitoring with Bravo capsule, and the PillCam.

10. **Why do I have symptoms if I have a normal endoscopy?**
    Seventy percent of patients with GERD have a normal endoscopy, which indicates they have non-erosive reflux disease (NERD). Acid reflux causes the symptoms you feel, but the mucosa (esophageal lining) is normal.

11. **What is the relationship between GERD and asthma?**
    The cause of asthma in at least 30 percent of patients is GERD. One should suspect GERD as the cause, especially when asthma develops during adulthood.

12. **Can GERD be diagnosed without a scope being inserted down my throat?**
    Yes. GERD, for the most part, is a clinical diagnosis based on symptoms. If further testing is needed to diagnose GERD or its complications and you do not want to have an endoscopy, there is a new technology, the PillCam, that can be used.

13. **What is Bravo?**
    Forty-eight-hour pH monitoring can be done using the Bravo capsule. This is done as a diagnostic test for GERD, especially in difficult situations, such as if the patient has atypical symptoms, the patient has the NERD variety of GERD, the diagnosis is not clear, and/or surgery is required. A gastroenterologist implants a capsule endoscopically in the esophagus, and this capsule remotely records the pH of the esophagus.

Frequently Asked Questions

14. **What does the PillCam do?**
    PillCam is a new technology used in diagnosing GERD or its complications noninvasively. The patient swallows a video camera the size of a pill that allows the physician to examine the inside of the esophagus.

15. **What treatments are available for GERD?**
    The treatment for GERD could include medications like antacids, H_2 blockers, prokinetic medications, or PPIs. In addition, a patient may need surgical treatment. Endoscopic treatment including endocinch, Stretta, and Enteryx are procedures that are still being studied.

16. **How long do I have to be on medications?**
    For the most part, treatment is long-term and symptoms return in a majority of patients if they stop medication. There is a subset of patients who can get by with on-demand therapy (as needed) and your physician will be able to tell you if you are one.

17. **What is the role of surgery in my treatment?**
    Surgery can now be done laparoscopically and is called the Nissen fundoplication. It is done in patients having breakthrough symptoms in spite of medication or patients who do not want to be on long-term medications, especially the younger population.

18. **Does Helicobacter pylori cause GERD?**
    No. H. Pylori are known to cause ulcers and inflammation of the stomach but not GERD.

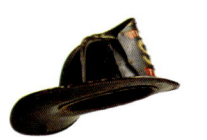

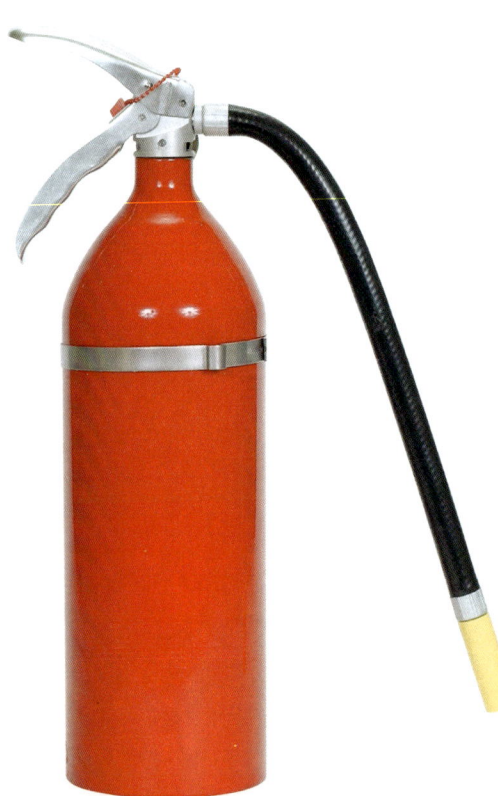

Use this glossary...

- For your own reference and understanding of terms related to GERD
- As an overview of important medical terms, procedures, and medications related to GERD
- To help you explain GERD concepts to others

Glossary

Barrett's esophagus — A pre-cancerous condition in which the squamous cells normally found in the esophagus change to columnar cells.

diaphragm — A muscle that separates the chest and abdomen.

diaphragmatic hiatus — An opening in the right side of the diaphragm, where the esophagus enters the stomach.

dilatation — The technique used to stretch or open a blocked portion of the esophagus.

dysphagia — Difficulty swallowing foods.

dysplasia — Pre-cancerous tissue changes.

EGD (esophagogastroduodenoscopy) — Using an endoscope to examine the upper digestive tract; commonly used in diagnosing GERD.

endocinch — Called "sewing," this is a procedure used to treat GERD with an endoscope. By placing sutures in the upper part of the stomach, the gastroesophageal junction is tightened.

endoscope — A flexible lighted instrument used to examine the internal areas of the body, including the upper GI tract. It is commonly used in the diagnosis of GERD.

Endoscopic mucosal resection — Surgery done with an endoscope for Barrett's esophagus with dysplasia; done only in selected centers in the United States. The specialist injects fluid under the lesion, thereby lifting it, and the lesion is then resected by a snare (an instrument that lassoes).

Enteryx — Called "stuffing," this is a procedure used to treat GERD utilizing an endoscope. It involves injecting the lower esophageal sphincter with a copolymer.

erosive esophagitis — Severe inflammation of the esophagus that causes development of erosions (mucosal breaks or "mini-ulcers" that are smaller than and not as deep as ulcers) and/or ulcers. This can cause anemia from slow blood loss or, on occasion, can cause severe hemorrhage. See chapter 4, "What Went Wrong?"

Glossary

esophageal adenocarcinoma — One of the most lethal cancers known to medicine.

esophageal motility study — This test determines if the esophagus is working correctly. A catheter is placed in the esophagus and the stomach. The patient is asked to swallow water and the esophageal pressures are recorded.

esophageal stricture — Narrowing of the esophagus

esophagitis — Esophageal inflammation. Can be mild or severe.

forty-eight-hour pH Bravo test — The only catheter-free pH monitoring system. With an endoscope, a miniature Bravo capsule is put in the esophagus. The capsule then tracks how often and how much acid comes back up into the esophagus.

Gatekeeper — This is an endoscopic procedure used outside the United States in the treatment of GERD. It has not been approved by the U.S. Food and Drug Administration.

H_2RAs or H_2 Blockers — These medications work by decreasing acidity; they do so by reducing the acid the stomach produces by blocking histamine$_2$ receptors on the parietal cells.

Helicobacter Pylori — A bacterium found in the stomach that damages tissue, causing ulcers to form.

hiatal hernia — A condition in which part of the upper stomach goes through the hiatus of the diaphragm into the chest.

laparascopy — Surgery that is done through several small incisions.

LES or lower esophageal sphincter — A muscle that acts as a "valve" where the esophagus enters the stomach.

Nissen fundoplication — A surgery for reflux in which the stomach is sewn around the esophagus. It is used to help acid reflux and to fix hiatal hernias.

odonophagia — Painful swallowing.

PPIs or proton pump inhibitors — Medications that decrease the gastric volume and acidity by blocking the acid production at the proton pump level. These medications are stronger than H_2RAs. See chapter 6, "Pills, Knife, or No More Spice" for a detailed explanation.

peristalsis — The wavelike contractions that move food down the esophagus into the stomach.

photodynamic therapy — A photosensitizing drug (called porfimer sodium) is injected intravenously; this drug stays in cancer cells longer than in other cells. Twenty-four to seventy-two hours later, the cancer cells in the esophagus are exposed to light through an endoscope, which activates the photosensitizer.

Glossary

When those photosensitizers are exposed to a particular wavelength of light, they emit oxygen, which kills nearby cells. In this case, the cancer cells are targeted.

phrenicoesophageal ligament — A ligament connecting the diaphragm and the LES (lower esophageal sphincter).

PillCam — A new technology in which a patient swallows a video camera the size of a pill. It enables physicians to examine the inside of the esophagus.

promotility or prokinetic drugs — These drugs work by increasing motility. Motility agents help by clearing the acid from the esophagus quickly and decreasing "contact time."

reflux esophagitis — Esophageal inflammation caused by GERD.

stretta (cooking) — This is one of the surgical ways to treat GERD. Radio frequency "cooking" of the LES and the upper stomach. When the area heals, scar tissue is formed, which as it heals causes the tissue to contract.

toupet — A surgical procedure used to treat GERD in which a surgeon does only a partial wrap of the upper portion of the stomach around the esophagus.

transient lower esophageal sphincter relaxation (TLESRs) — A transient relaxation of the lower esophageal sphincter that happens naturally in everyone, particularly after eating, to release air and gas in the stomach. But in patients with GERD, TLESRs can last up to thirty seconds and may not be associated with a swallow, causing acid reflux.

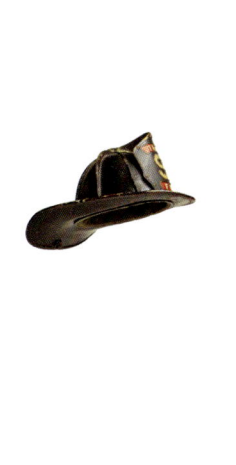

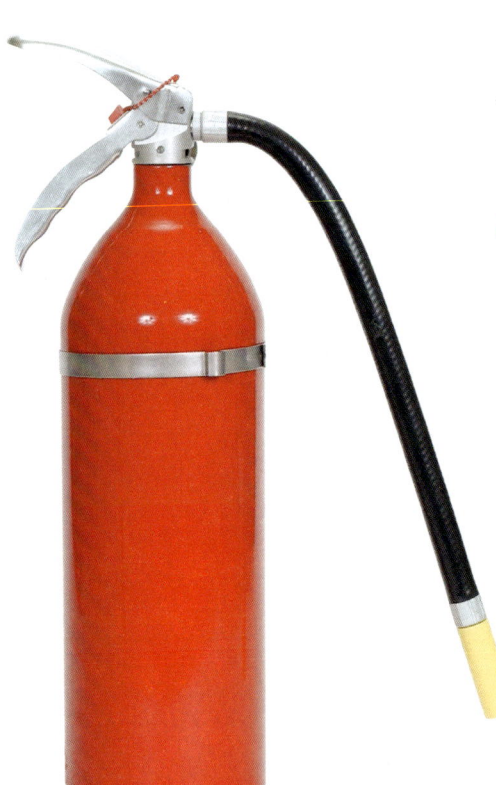

In this appendix...
- Staples to keep in your pantry if you suffer from GERD
- Eating out when you have GERD
- GERD-friendly recipes

Recipes Amenable to GERD Sufferers

Heartburn can be greatly exacerbated by eating the wrong foods. The challenge for those suffering from this symptom is figuring out which foods are the wrong ones.

Unfortunately, although it is possible to generalize about foods that tend to aggravate heartburn, individuals vary in their reactions to those foods. For instance, raw onions often cause heartburn, but for some people, cooked onions are fine. It may be difficult to identify which food it is that causes the problem. Was it heavy cream in the fettuccine Alfredo or the lettuce in the salad that preceded the meal?

Experiment to determine which foods aggravate your GERD symptoms. Try the fettuccine without the salad, for instance. Or

Spurn the Burn

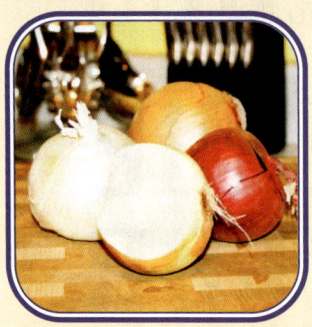

FIGURE 26
Onions may exacerbate GERD...

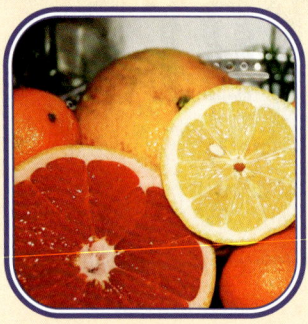

FIGURE 27
... as do citrus fruits.

leave the cheese off your sandwich or the onions out of your chili. Add those foods back into your diet one at a time, and it will become clear which items cause the most problems.

That said, there are many foods that typically cause heartburn, and you can learn to cook in a manner that will help keep your symptoms to a minimum. Some people with minor symptoms are even able to control their heartburn by eating a particular diet.

Watch out for fats, chocolate, caffeine, oils, alcohol, and citrus products, as they typically cause problems. Pat Baird, dietician with the National Heartburn Alliance, has numerous recommendations for handling your diet on that organization's Web site, www.heartburnalliance.org, and we've reprinted some here. For additional recipes and diet advice, see Elaine Magee's book, *Tell Me What to Eat If I Have Acid Reflux*.

Keep These Items Handy in Your Cupboard

- **Grains:** Try to purchase whole grains instead of refined grains whenever possible. Be sure to store them in an airtight container after opening. Some that seem fine for most people

Recipes Amenable to Gerd Sufferers

include brown rice, basmati rice, short-grain rice, polenta (instant and regular), quick-cooking oats, quick-cooking grits, and stone-ground cornmeal.

> The National Heartburn Alliance offers a Personal Reflux Record to help you track and record what foods cause you the most trouble. For more information, visit its Web site at www.heartburnalliance.org and go to the section titled "Food for Thought."

- **Pasta:** Be sure to prepare these with a light "broth-type" sauce (not tomato-based or high-fat). Perk up the dish with herbs like basil and tarragon. Try bow-tie, linguine, fettuccine, spaghetti, penne, orzo (rice-shaped pasta), and rigatoni.

- **Beans, peas, and lentils:** All these items provide a good source of vegetable protein, B vitamins, and minerals such as calcium and iron. They are also an excellent source of fiber. Keep both dried and canned varieties on your shelf, and toss them into soups, salads, pasta, and casserole dishes. Try red kidney beans, black beans, white kidney beans, split peas (yellow, green), navy beans, scarlet runners, lentils, and chickpeas.

- **Oils:** Use oils in moderation. The darker oils (like sesame) have wonderful flavor, and a little goes a long way in adding good taste and enjoyment to dishes. Keep cooking-oil sprays in the cupboard. This cuts down on extra fat and the different varieties can add flavor, too. Try extra-virgin olive, sesame (light and dark), walnut, and canola oils.

- **Vinegars:** These can be problem items for severe heartburn sufferers because of the acid content. However, cider vinegar and rice vinegar often are tolerated better by many people, and both add nice flavor to food. Use other vinegars with discretion if there hasn't been a problem with them in the past.

- **Condiments and Canned Goods:** Most people with heartburn can eat mustard, and some can handle ketchup (in small amounts) fairly well. These are handy items to perk up recipes and provide quick add-ons to a meal. Try soy sauce, chicken and vegetable broth, dried mushrooms, reduced-fat mayonnaise, reduced-fat peanut butter, fat-free salad dressings, dried fruits, fruit spreads, canned fruits, canned vegetables, and canned (and dried) soups.

- **Spices and Herbs:** Keep lots of dried spices and herbs on the shelf. They are generally less likely to promote heartburn — though each individual's system will respond differently. Dried or dehydrated forms of onion and garlic are more user-friendly than fresh! Try ground cinnamon, ground mace, garlic powder, basil, thyme, tarragon, coriander, dill, onion powder and dried onion pieces, dill, and parsley.

    There are several spices that are generally irritating to the gastric (stomach) lining and are especially troublesome for heartburn sufferers. The spices listed following may be troublesome for some sufferers but pose no problem for others. The best advice is to listen to one's own body. This spice group includes black pepper, mint, crushed red pepper

Recipes Amenable to Gerd Sufferers

flakes, cloves, Tabasco sauce, mustard seeds, fresh garlic (raw or cooked), chili powder, and curry powder.

Eating Out

Dining out can be a challenge because it can be difficult to know what is in every menu item and to choose something that you're confident won't cause heartburn.

Identifying what your personal trigger foods are will help you eliminate obvious items. The challenge is that most restaurant foods tend to be high in fat. Fat takes longer to digest, so food stays in the stomach longer and has a greater likelihood of causing problems, according to Baird. Restaurant portions also tend to be larger than recommended serving sizes. This increases pressure in the stomach and may cause acidic stomach contents to splash back into the esophagus.

When ordering at a restaurant, avoid cream and tomato sauces, oil-based salad dressings, anything deep-fat fried, spicy foods, rich and heavy desserts, and, of course, anything containing your personal triggers. Don't

Questions to ask when dining out:
- How is the dish prepared?
- Can my menu selection be grilled or broiled instead of fried or sautéed?
- Does this dish come with a high-fat gravy or sauce that could be served on the side?
- Could I split an entrée with a friend rather than order a large meal on my own?

Source: National Heartburn Alliance

~

It's wise to avoid frying, deep-frying, and sautéing whenever possible. In lieu of frying or sautéing, try steaming vegetables, seafood, or poultry using broths, juices, water, wine, or dry vermouth. (Note: Cooking with alcohol does not tend to exacerbate heartburn because the alcohol cooks off as the recipe is heated.) This can be done on top of the stove or in the microwave in a covered container. With some foods like chicken or potatoes, roasting achieves an effect and flavor similar to deep-frying.

Source: National Heartburn Alliance

Spurn the Burn

forget to consider what you're drinking; caffeinated beverages and alcohol tend to cause heartburn.

Following are some recipes, developed by Baird for the National Heartburn Alliance, that will give you tasty options as you plan your weekly menu.

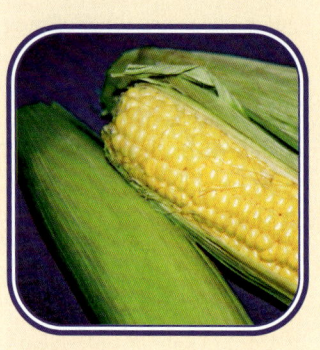

FIGURE 28
Corn

Whole Wheat Corn Muffins

These light, whole-grain muffins are the perfect way to start the day or to keep tucked in the freezer for a handy snack. They contain far less fat than packaged muffins, and that's always a plus for heartburn sufferers.

Makes 12 muffins

> 1 cup stone-ground yellow corn meal
> ⅔ cup all-purpose flour
> ⅓ cup whole-wheat flour
> 1 teaspoon baking powder
> 1 teaspoon baking soda
> ½ teaspoon salt
> 1 cup nonfat plain yogurt
> 1 egg
> ¼ cup vegetable oil*
> ¼ cup honey
> 1 teaspoon vanilla extract

Recipes Amenable to Gerd Sufferers

1. Preheat oven to 400° F. Lightly spray a 12-cup muffin pan with nonstick cooking spray; set aside.

2. In a large bowl whisk together the corn meal, both flours, baking powder, baking soda, and salt.

3. In a medium bowl whisk together the yogurt, egg, oil, honey, and vanilla. Make a well in the center of the flour mixture. Pour in the yogurt mixture; and stir until just combined (do not overmix). Spoon the batter into the prepared pan. Bake for 18 to 20 minutes, or until golden brown. Transfer the muffins to a wire rack to cool.

* Use the same cup to measure the honey without washing after measuring the oil. The honey will glide out of the cup.

Nutrient Information Per Serving:

Calories 151 **Carbohydrate** 22g **Protein** 4g
Fat 5g **Sodium** 240mg **Cholesterol** 18mg

· ·

Bow-Tie Pasta with Peas and Ham

This easy pasta recipe uses a "broth-type" sauce rather than a tomato-based one, which can aggravate heartburn. Buy frozen vegetables in bags so you can measure what you need and keep the remainder frozen. Feel free to substitute cooked chicken or turkey, leftover seafood, or lean beef in this recipe. Fresh herbs, when they're available, always enhance the overall flavor of the dish.

Spurn the Burn

Makes 4 servings

- 12 ounces bow-tie pasta, uncooked
- 2 tablespoons olive oil
- ½ teaspoon garlic powder
- 1 14.5 ounce can reduced-sodium chicken broth
- ¾ teaspoon dried basil *or* thyme, crumbled (or 1 tablespoon fresh)
- 1 cup frozen "petite" peas
- 4 ounces low-sodium boiled ham, thinly sliced and cut into ½" strips
- Grated Parmesan cheese, optional

1. Cook the pasta according to package directions.

2. In a medium saucepan, heat the oil over medium heat. Stir in garlic powder and cook for 15 seconds. Pour in the broth; stir in the basil (or thyme), and cook for 3 minutes, or until just boiling.

3. Place the peas in a large colander. Drain the pasta directly over the peas. Return the pasta and peas to the pan; and pour in the broth. Turn burner heat to medium-high; add the ham, and toss well to combine. Cook for about 2 minutes, or until piping hot.

4. To serve, ladle pasta into serving bowls, and serve with grated cheese, if desired.

Recipes Amenable to Gerd Sufferers

Nutrient Information Per Serving:
Calories 444   Carbohydrate 21g   Protein 4g
Fat 4g   Sodium 240mg   Cholesterol 18mg

• •

Herbed Orzo Salad with Corn

This simple salad, made with corn and fresh basil, is just right for summer menus. Orzo is small pasta that resembles rice. This side dish is versatile and heartburn friendly because it's low in fat; it's loaded with flavor yet doesn't contain any irritating spices. It quickly turns into a main dish when tossed with cooked chicken, grilled salmon, or any other cooked meat.

Makes 4 servings

- 1 cup orzo
- 1 cup fresh corn niblets *or* frozen, defrosted corn
- ¼ cup sliced (jar) pimento
- 3 tablespoons chopped fresh basil
- 2 tablespoons white Balsamic *or* apple cider vinegar
- 1 tablespoon olive oil
- ½ teaspoon salt

1. Cook orzo according to package directions. Drain thoroughly and transfer to a large bowl. Stir in the corn, pimento, basil, vinegar, oil, and salt; toss thoroughly to combine. Adjust seasoning, if desired. Serve at room temperature.

Spurn the Burn

* Note: If preparing this recipe ahead, cover and refrigerate. Before serving, let stand at room temperature for about 1 hour to remove the chill. Stir thoroughly and serve.

Nutrient Information Per Serving:

Calories 230   Carbohydrate 40g   Protein 7g
Fat 5g   Sodium 300mg   Cholesterol 0mg

- -

Marinated Lamb Loins

Lamb is a tasty alternative to beef. Cuts of lamb, like the loin, are low in fat, which can be a good choice for heartburn sufferers. Orange juice gives the marinade a sweet, fresh taste and is not an irritant since so little is used. Rosemary is one of the best herbs to use when cooking lamb, and it perks up the recipe.

Makes 4 servings

> 1 pound lamb loin
> ⅓ cup orange juice
> 2 tablespoons packed brown sugar
> 1 tablespoon olive oil
> 1 teaspoon dried rosemary, crumbled
> ½ teaspoon salt

1. In a small bowl, whisk together the orange juice, brown sugar, oil, rosemary, and salt.

Recipes Amenable to Gerd Sufferers

2. Place the lamb in a shallow glass casserole dish, and pour the mixture over the top. Turn the lamb over several times to coat. Cover the casserole, and refrigerate for about 2 hours, turning occasionally.

3. Preheat grill (or oven) to 375°F.

4. Remove the lamb from the marinade. Discard any unused marinade. Place on preheated grill (if roasting, place it on a baking sheet). Cook for about 15 minutes, or until desired doneness. Let stand for 5 minutes. Slice the loin diagonally into ½-inch slices and serve.

Nutrient Information Per Serving:
Calories 120   **Carbohydrate** 4g   **Protein** 13g
Fat 6g   **Sodium** 185mg   **Cholesterol** 40mg

· ·

Grilled Marinated Flank Steak

Few people realize that flank steak is one of the leanest cuts of beef. This recipe has flavor without the fat, and fat is a major culprit in creating heartburn. Guests will love it, too.

Makes 4 servings

> ¼ cup balsamic vinegar
> 2 tablespoons reduced sodium-soy sauce
> 2 tablespoons honey

Spurn the Burn

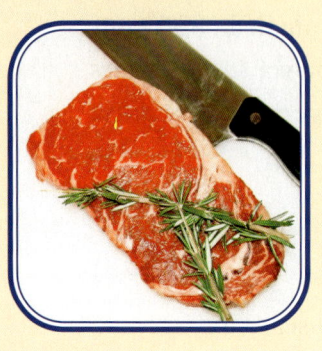

FIGURE 29
Flank Steak

2 medium shallots, thinly sliced
2 teaspoons fresh chopped rosemary *or* 1 teaspoon dried rosemary
1 ½ teaspoons dry mustard
1 ¼ pounds flank steak
Salt to taste

1. In a 13 x 9 x 2-inch glass baking dish combine the vinegar, soy sauce, honey, shallots, rosemary, and mustard until combined, using a fork or whisk.

2. Place the steak on top, and press meat lightly to coat with marinade. Turn and press again. Cover and refrigerate for at least 2 hours, turning occasionally.

3. Prepare grill to medium-hot coals or medium setting, or preheat broiler. Remove the meat from marinade; discard marinade. Grill 4 to 6 minutes on each side (for medium-rare), or until desired doneness. Transfer steak to cutting board; sprinkle lightly with salt. Let stand for 5 minutes. Cut diagonally across the grain into thin slices. Arrange on a platter and serve.

Nutrient Information Per Serving:
Calories 224   Carbohydrate 4g   Protein 27g
Fat 10g   Sodium 166mg   Cholesterol 67mg

Recipes Amenable to Gerd Sufferers

Roasted Sweet Potatoes and Summer Vegetables

Prepare this delightful combination of potatoes and vegetables on the grill or in the oven. They can be made ahead and served at room temperature, or reheated when you're ready to eat. Sweet Vidalia onions are easy on your tummy — especially when they're roasted — so former onion eaters may tolerate them quite well. Sweet potatoes are so rich in nutrients everyone should eat them whenever possible. Feel free, however, to substitute your favorite potato in this recipe.

Makes 4 servings

> 2 medium sweet potatoes, scrubbed and cut into $\frac{1}{2}$-inch pieces
> 1 medium Vidalia onion, thinly sliced
> 1 medium zucchini, cut into 1-inch pieces (about 12 ounces)
> 1 medium yellow summer squash, cut into 1-inch pieces (about 12 ounces)
> 1 tablespoon + 1 teaspoon extra-virgin olive oil
> 1 tablespoon chopped fresh thyme *or* 2 teaspoons dried, crumbled thyme
> Salt to taste

1. Prepare grill to medium-hot coals or medium setting, or preheat oven to 425° F.

2. In a shallow baking pan, combine the vegetables, olive oil, and thyme; toss until thoroughly combined. Cook on

preheated grill, or in preheated oven, for about 35 minutes, or until vegetables are tender and lightly browned, stirring occasionally.

Nutrient Information Per Serving:

Calories 147   Carbohydrate 24g   Protein 3g
Fat 5g   Sodium 14mg   Cholesterol 0mg

• •

Spinach Stuffed Sole

This colorful entrée will please your sweetheart in more ways than one. Fish is highly regarded as a heart-healthy food. This recipe is low in fat, packed with flavor and about as heartburn friendly as it gets.

Makes 4 servings

- 1 10-ounce package frozen chopped spinach, thawed and squeezed of excess liquid
- 1 2-ounce jar sliced pimento, drained and divided
- 2 ounces feta cheese, crumbled
- 2 tablespoons low-fat mayonnaise
- $\frac{1}{8}$ teaspoon ground nutmeg
- 4 six-ounce fillets of sole *or* flounder
- 2 teaspoons butter, cut into 4 pieces
- paprika

Recipes Amenable to Gerd Sufferers

1. Preheat oven to 400° F. Lightly spray a baking sheet with non-stick cooking spray.

2. In a medium bowl combine the spinach, cheese, mayonnaise, nutmeg, and half the pimento; use a fork to blend. Place an even amount of the mixture on half of each fillet; fold other half over to enclose mixture. Place fillets on prepared baking sheet; top each with a piece of the butter. Sprinkle lightly with paprika. Bake for 15 minutes, or until fish flakes when tested with a fork.

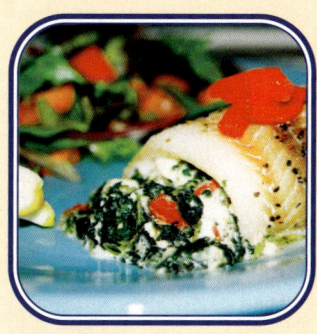

FIGURE 30
Stuffed Sole

3. To serve, place fish on serving plates, and top with a few pieces of the remaining pimentos.

4. Serve immediately.

Nutrient Information Per Serving:

Calories 240　　**Carbohydrate** 4g　　**Protein** 36g
Fat 8g　　**Sodium** 380mg　　**Cholesterol** 110mg

Spurn the Burn

Angel Food Cake

This is the consummate guiltless dessert: It's fat-free and cholesterol-free. Heartburn sufferers, weight watchers, and anyone who loves dessert is bound to ask for seconds on this. A big, plump strawberry thinly sliced (not all the way through) and fanned out makes an attractive garnish. Having the egg whites at room temperature is important for them to beat up high and fluffy — allow 20 to 30 minutes for this.

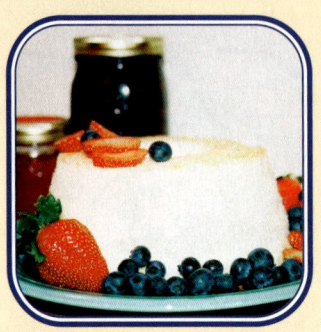

FIGURE 31
Angel food cake with fruit

Makes 12 servings

- 1¼ cups superfine sugar, divided
- 1 cup sifted cake flour
- 12 large egg whites, at room temperature
- 1 teaspoon cream of tartar
- ½ teaspoon salt
- 2 teaspoons vanilla extract

1. Preheat oven to 375° F.

2. In a medium bowl whisk together ¾ cup of the sugar and the cake flour; set aside.

3. In a large bowl, using an electric mixer at medium speed, beat the egg whites until thick and foamy. Increase the

Recipes Amenable to Gerd Sufferers

speed to high, and add the cream of tartar, salt, and vanilla. Beat until soft peaks form; sprinkle the remaining sugar gradually over the top of the batter, while beating. Continue to beat until stiff and glossy. Do not overbeat.

4. In three batches, gently (and quickly) fold the flour mixture into the egg white mixture, using a rubber spatula, slotted spoon, or large balloon whisk. Pour the batter into an ungreased 10-inch tube pan with removable sides; use a narrow metal spatula or sharp knife to cut through the batter, eliminate any air pockets. Bake for 30 to 35 minutes, or until a tester inserted the center comes out clean.

5. Invert the cake over a funnel, or narrow bottle to cool. Run a long, thin knife around the side of the cake, and release the sides of the pan.

Nutrient Information Per Serving:

Calories 130   **Carbohydrate** 28g   **Protein** 4g
Fat 0g   **Sodium** 190mg   **Cholesterol** 0mg

Wild Mushroom Stuffing

No one will realize this stuffing is not loaded with fat and cholesterol. The wonderful flavors of the mushrooms make a stuffing you'll be proud to serve throughout the holiday season.

Makes about 10 cups (ten 1-cup servings)

Spurn the Burn

1 pound loaf unsliced sourdough bread, cut or torn into 1-inch cubes
2 tablespoons vegetable oil
2 cups chopped celery (with leaves)
½ pound assorted wild mushrooms (such as shiitake or cremini), sliced
½ pound white mushrooms, sliced
½ cup chopped flat-leaf (Italian) parsley
1 cup egg substitute
1 cup reduced-sodium chicken broth
1 ½ teaspoons dried thyme
½ teaspoon salt
½ teaspoon ground nutmeg

1. In a 15 x 10 x 2 baking pan, arrange bread cubes in an even layer. Set aside for several hours to dry, tossing occasionally.

2. Preheat oven to 325° F.

3. In a large nonstick skillet, heat the oil for 1 minute over medium heat. Add the celery and cook for 2 minutes, stirring occasionally. Add the mushrooms, and cook 3 to 5 minutes longer, or until the mushrooms are softened and the celery is tender. Stir in the parsley; cook 1 minute longer. Set aside to cool slightly.

4. In a large mixing bowl combine the reserved bread and mushroom mixture (with any accumulated juices), tossing well to combine. Add the egg substitute, broth, thyme, salt,

Recipes Amenable to Gerd Sufferers

and nutmeg; stir thoroughly to blend. (Add more broth or water if you prefer very moist stuffing.)

5. Spray the roasting pan with nonstick cooking spray. Spoon in the stuffing and smooth to make an even layer. Cover with aluminum foil and bake at 325° F for 25 minutes. Remove foil and bake 15 minutes longer, or until top is crisp.

· ·

Roasted Onion and Shallot Gravy

The sweet Vidalia onion add both richness and flavor to this virtually fat-free gravy. Shallots replace troublesome garlic and add depth as well. This gravy freezes beautifully, so you may find yourself making it all year long to have on hand for last-minute meals.

Makes about 6 cups (twelve ½-cup servings)

- 2 tablespoons olive oil or canola oil
- 2 large Vidalia onions, thinly sliced
- 2 large shallots, thinly sliced
- ½ teaspoon salt
- 2 cans (14.5 ounces each) reduced-sodium chicken broth, divided
- ½ teaspoon dried thyme, crushed
- 1 teaspoon Gravy Master

1. In a large nonstick skillet, heat the oil for 1 minute over medium heat. Add the onions and shallots, and cook for 2

minutes, stirring frequently. Reduce heat to low and cook for 15 to 20 minutes, or until the vegetables are golden brown, stirring occasionally. Sprinkle with salt, and set aside to cool slightly.

2. Transfer the onion mixture and ½ cup of the broth to a food processor, and process until smooth. With motor running, gradually pour in about 1 ½ cups of the broth (or whatever the food processor will handle without overflowing), and process until thoroughly combined.

3. Transfer the gravy to a large saucepan. Add the remaining broth, thyme, and Gravy Master. Heat just to boiling over medium heat; adjust seasoning and color to taste. Serve immediately.

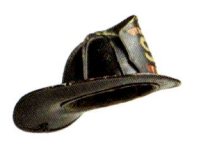

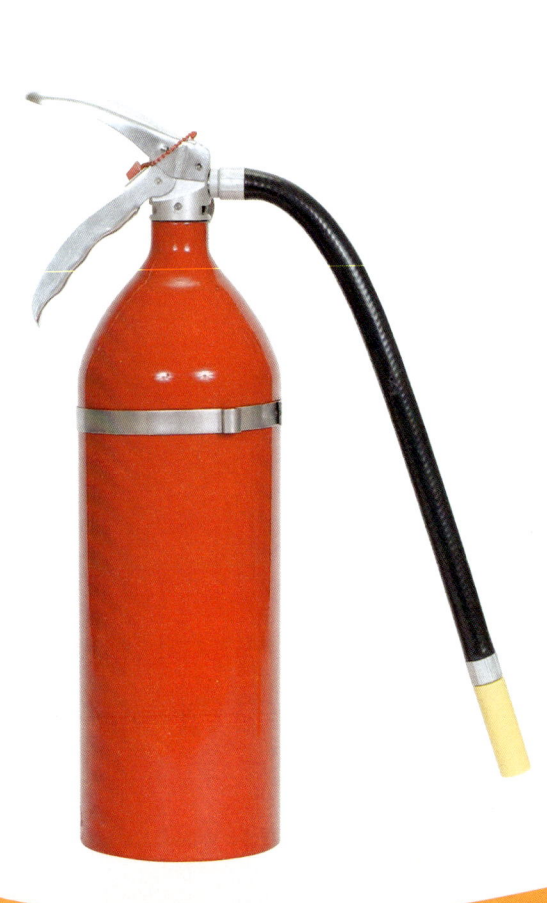

Recommended Websites

National Heartburn Alliance
www.heartburnalliance.com

Midwest Heartburn Clinic
www.midwestheartburnclinic.com

The American Gastroenterological Association
www.gastro.org

American College of Gastroenterology
www.acg.gi.org

American Society for Gastrointestinal Endoscopy
www.asge.org

American Dietetic Association
www.eatright.org

AcipHex (rabeprazole sodium)
www.aciphex.com

Nexium, the Healing Purple Pill
www.purplepill.com

Prevacid (lansoprazole)
www.prevacid.com

Protonix (pantoprazole sodium)
www.protonix.com

Astra Pharmaceuticals' GERD Information Resource Center
www.gerd.com

Prilosec OTC
www.prilosecOTC.com

The Recipe Doctor, Elaine Magee, MPH, RD
www.recipedoctor.com

Kansas Medical Clinic Professional Association
www.kmcpa.com

Recommended Websites

Given Imaging
www.givenimaging.com

Medtronic, Inc.
www.medtronic.com
www.bravophtesting.org

Winning the Hepatitis C Battle
www.hepcbattle.com

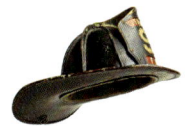

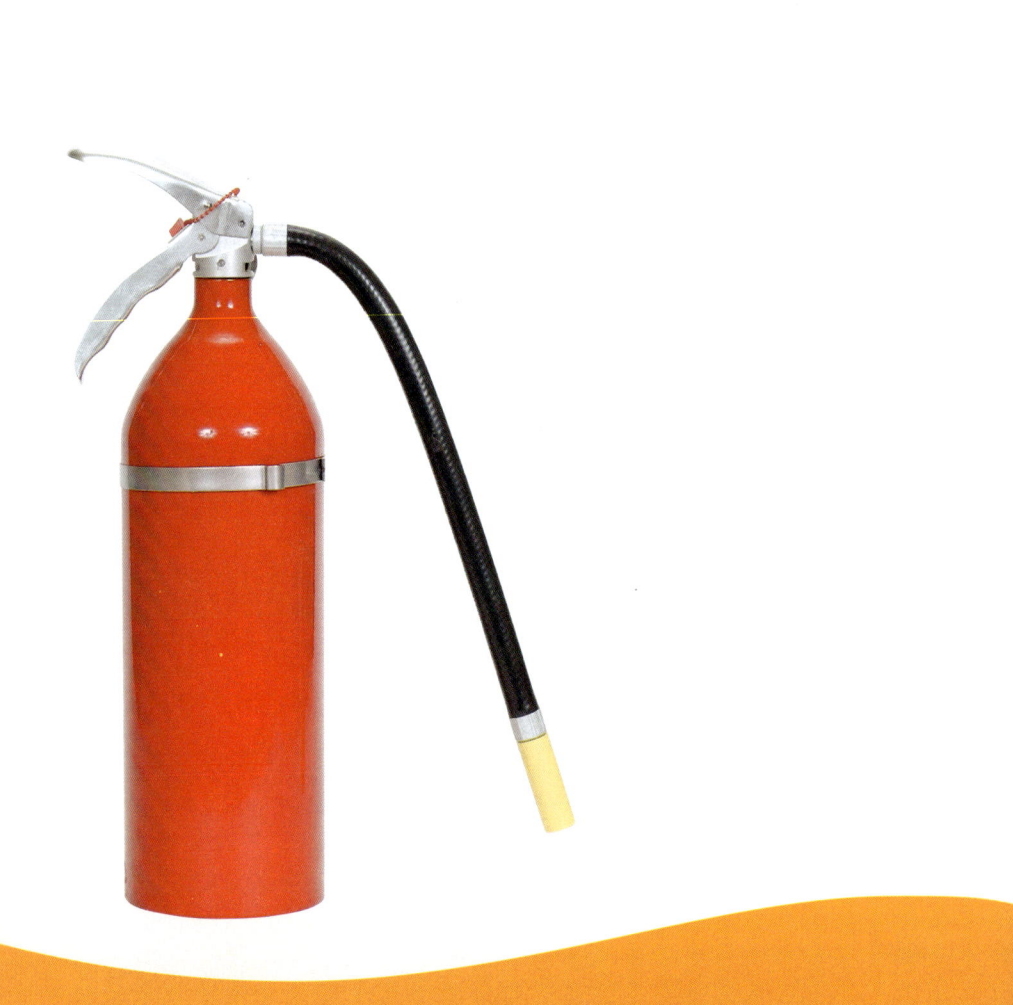

Index

Page numbers followed by f refer to figures.

A

Acetylcholine receptor, 57
Acetylcholine receptor pathway, 20
Acid, stomach
   alternative treatments for, 71–73
   turmeric for, 73
Acid suppression therapy, 57–60
Aciphex, xxviii, 59
Age. *See also* Elderly patients
and GERD, 1
   and incidence of Barrett's esophagus, 30
   and incidence of erosive esophagitis, 28–29
   and severity of symptoms *vs.* disease, 79–80

"Agitated esophagus," and Aloe vera juice, 73
Alcohol
   as aggravating factor, 15, 54, 104, 107
   cooking with, 107
   and hypotensive LES, 22–23
   and sour burps, 74
Alginic acid, 56
Allergies
   licorice as alternative treatment for, 72
   ragweed, and chamomile, 70–71
Aloe vera juice
   and "agitated esophagus," 73
   as alternative treatment, 73

Alternative and complementary
   treatments, 69–75
   clinical studies on, 71–72
      controversial nature of, 71
   consulting physicians on, 70
      especially licorice, 72
   FDA non-regulation of, 70
   interaction of herbs with prescription medications, 70, 72
   National Health Interview Survey on, 69
   side effects of, 70, 72
   spending on, 69
Aluminum-based calcium carbonate, in antacids, 55
American Botanical Council, on alternative medicines, 70
Anemia
   and erosive esophagitis, 28
   and esophageal cancer, 35
Angel food cake, recipe for, 118–119
Angelica root, European (Angelica archangelica), as alternative treatment, 75
Anise, as alternative treatment, 75
Antacids, 55–56, 91
   first-person account of, 54
   and pregnancy, 78
   side effects of, 54–55
Anti-cholinergic medications, as aggravating factor, 16
Antidepressants, tricyclic, as aggravating factor, 16
Anxiety, and promotility drugs, 56

Apple juice, and stomach acid, 71
Artichoke, as alternative treatment, 75
Aspirin
   as aggravating factor, 16
   and EGD, 42
Asteraceae (ragweed family), allergy to, and chamomile, 70–71
Asthma
   in case study, 6–7
   and GERD in children, 79
   as symptom, 13, 88, 90
Axid, xxviii, 58
   and pregnancy, 58

B

Babies, and GERD, 79
Baclofen, 56–57
Bacteria, and GERD. *See* Helicobacter pylori
Bad breath (halitosis), as symptom, 13–14
Baird, Pat, 104, 107–108
Barium esophagram/upper gastrointestinal series test, for diagnosis of GERD vs. hiatal hernia, 46–47
Barrett, Norman Rupert, 30, 30f
Barrett's esophagus, 28–33, 31f, 32f
   in case study, 2
   definition of, 30, 95
   and dysplasia, 29–30
   and EGD, 41
   and hiatal hernia, 30–31
   prevalence of, 29

Index

and risk of esophageal cancer, xxvi, 28, 35, 88
and Stretta procedure, 61
testing for, 39
treatment of, 31–32
Basil, as alternative treatment, 75
Beans, in GERD-friendly diet, 105
Bed, elevated, *vs.* pillows, 53–54
Belching. *See also* Sour burps
inability to belch, after surgery, 65
as symptom, 14
Beta$_2$ agonists, as aggravating factor, 16
Beta blockers, as aggravating factor, 16
Bethanecol, 56
Biaxin, interactions with PPIs, 60
Bicarbonate, in saliva, and nocturnal reflux, 11
Biopsy, and EGD, 41
Birth control pills, as aggravating factor, 16
"Bitter digestive stimulants," as alternative treatment, 71
Bitters, stomach, 74
artichoke as, 75
Blessed thistle, as alternative treatment, 71
Blood in stool, and GERD screening, 40
Blood loss, and erosive esophagitis, 28
Blood-thinning agents, and EGD, 42
Boldo, as alternative treatment, 75

Bone-density medications, as aggravating factor, 16
Bravo pH Monitoring System, xxix, 40, 44–46, 45*f*, 84, 90
in case study, 5
charts of results, 46*f*, 47*f*
first-person account of, 48
as pre-surgery test, 63
Breath, bad (halitosis), as symptom, 13–14
Bricanyl, as aggravating factor, 16
Bronchial infections, recurrent, as symptom, 13, 88
Bronchitis, alternative treatments for, 72
Burps, sour. *See* Sour burps

C

Caffeine, as aggravating factor, 15, 89, 107
Cake, angel food, recipe for, 118–119
Calcium, and chamomile, 70
Calcium channel blockers
as aggravating factor, 16
and hypotensive LES, 22–23
Calendula, as alternative treatment, 72
Camomile. *See* Chamomile
Cancer of the esophagus. *See* Esophageal adenocarcinoma
Canned food, in GERD-friendly diet, 106
Carafate, 60
Caraway, as alternative treatment, 71

Cardamom, as alternative treatment, 75
Cardizem, as aggravating factor, 16
Carminative medicines, 71, 75
   as alternative treatment, 71, 75
   and gas, 71
Carrot juice, and stomach acid, 71
Case studies, 1–7
Catheter
   for pH measurement, 44
   in pre-surgery motility test, 63
Catnip
   as alternative treatment, 72
   and digestion, 72
Catnip tea, as alternative treatment, 73
Cells
   columnar, in stomach, 15, 29–30
   parietal, in stomach, and hydrochloric acid, 10, 20, 57
   squamous, in esophagus, 15, 29–30
Centaurium
   as alternative treatment, 74
   and pregnancy, 74
Chamomile (Matricaria recutita)
   as alternative treatment, 70–72
   American Botanical Council and, 70
   calming properties of, 70
   ragweed allergies and, 70–71
Chest pain, as symptom of GERM, 88
   in case study, 4
   first-person account of, 9
   mistaken for heart attack, 4, 9, 12–13
Children, and GERD, 79
Chocolate
   as aggravating factor, 15, 53, 89, 104
   and hypotensive LES, 22–23
Choking, as symptom
   in case study, 2
   in infants, 79
Chrysanthemums, allergy to, and chamomile, 70–71
Cimetidine, 58
   and gynecomastia (enlarged breasts), 58
   and impotence, 58
Cinnamon, as alternative treatment, 75
Cisapride, 56–57
Citrus juices, as aggravating factor, 15, 53, 89, 104
Clearing throat, need for, as symptom, 13
Cline, Jim, case study of, 5, 5f
Cloves, as alternative treatment, 75
Coffee
   as aggravating factor, 15, 53, 89, 107
   in case study, 2
   and sour burps, 74
Cola drinks (caffeinated), as aggravating factor, 15, 53, 89, 107
Colds, licorice as alternative treatment for, 72
Complementary medicine. See Al-

Index

ternative and complementary treatments
Condiments, in GERD-friendly diet, 106
Constipation, as side effect of antacids, 54–55
"Cooking" (surgical procedure). See Stretta procedure
Coriander, as alternative treatment, 75
Corn muffins, whole wheat, recipe for, 108–109
Cough, chronic, as symptom, 13, 88
  in case studies, 3–4, 5, 6–7
  in infants, 79
Coumadin
  and EGD, 42
  interactions with PPIs, 60
Cramping, and carminative medications, 71
Cream sauces, as aggravating factor, 107
Crying, and GERD in infants, 79

D

Defibrillator, implantable, and Bravo pH Monitoring System, 45
Delayed esophageal clearance, 23
Delayed gastric emptying, 23
Demerol, as aggravating factor, 16
Demulcent (soothing, coating agent), licorice as, 72
Dental decay, 14*f*
  as symptom, 13, 88
Depression, and promotility drugs, 56
Dessert, rich or heavy, as aggravating factor, 107
Diabetes
  and delayed gastric emptying, 23
  and EGD, 42
  and licorice as alternative treatment, 72–73
Diagnosis of GERD, 39–48, 89
Diaphragm, 22, 95
Diaphragmatic hiatus, 21, 95
Diarrhea
  and H_2RAs, 58
  and PPIs, 59
  as side effect of antacids, 54–55
Diet, low-fat and high-protein, 53
Digestion. *See also* Indigestion
  and catnip, 72
  and chamomile, 70
  and chewable papaya enzyme tablets, 75
  and dill seeds, 73
  and ginger, 70
  and papaya or papaya seeds, 75
  and pineapple, 75
  and relief chi herbal treatment, 74
  and stomach bitters, 74
  and turmeric, 73
Digestive system, 20*f*
  components of, 19, 20*f*
Digoxin, interactions with PPIs, 60
Dilatation, esophageal

definition of, 95
 for dysphagia after surgery, 64–65
 for esophageal stricture, 34
 first-person account of, 34
Dill and dill seeds, as alternative treatment, 73, 75
Dining out, and GERD-friendly foods, 107–108
Domperidone, 56–57
Drowsiness, and promotility drugs, 56
Drugs. *See* Medications
Duodenum, and EGD, 41
Dysphagia (difficulty swallowing)
 after surgery, 64
 definition of, 95
 and esophageal cancer, 35
 and esophageal stricture, 33–34
 and GERD diagnosis, 40
 as sign of complications, 11
 as symptom, 11, 88
Dysplasia, 32*f*
 and aggressive treatment, 31
 and Barrett's esophagus, 29–30
 definition of, 96
 low-grade *vs.* high-grade, 30

E

Ear infections, and GERD in children, 79
Echinacea, allergy to, and chamomile, 70–71
EGD (esophagogastroduodenoscopy), endoscopy, 40, 41–42. *See also* Endoscope
 in case studies, 2, 5, 6
 definition of, 96
 and erosive *vs.* non-erosive GERD, 14
 fear of, xxvii, xxviii, 43–44
 first-person account of, 41
 gastroscope and, 41, 41*f*
 before surgery, 63
Elavil, as aggravating factor, 16
Elderly patients. *See also* Age
 and decreased resistance of esophageal mucosa, 24
 and GERD, 79–80
Elm, slippery. *See* Slippery elm
Endocinch procedure (surgical), 61, 84, 91
 definition of, 96
Endoscope. *See also* EGD
 definition of, 96
 in PDT, 32
 and surgical procedures, 61–62
Endoscopic management, 61–62
Endoscopic mucosal resection, 32, 35, 84
 definition of, 96
Endoscopic procedures (laparoscopic surgery), 61–62
Endoscopy. *See* EGD
Enteryx, injection with (surgical procedure), 61, 84, 91
 definition of, 96
Enzymes
 digestive

Index

and "bitter digestive stimulants," 71
and stomach bitters, 74
plant, in relief chi herbal treatment, 74
Epigastric pain. See Pain, epigastric
Erosions, esophageal
  definition of, 28
  and esophageal stricture, 33
Erythromycin, 56–57
Esomeprazole, 58–59
Esophageal adenocarcinoma (cancer of the esophagus), 32f, 34–36, 35f
  definition of, 97
  first-person account of, 35
  increased incidence of, xxvi–xxvii, 34
  lethality of, 34, 35–36, 88
Esophageal motility study, 46, 47–48
  definition of, 97
Esophageal stricture, 33–34, 34f, 88
  definition of, 97
  and dysphagia, 33–34
  and odonophagia, 33–34
Esophagitis, 15f
  definition of, 97
  erosive, 88
    definition of, 96
    vs. ulcerative, 28
  grading of (1-4 or A-D), 14, 28, 29f

incidence vs. gender, race, age, 28–29
non-erosive. See NERD (non-erosive esophagitis)
reflux, definition of, 99
Esophagus, 15f, 19, 20–22, 20f, 21f, 24f
  "agitated," and Aloe vera juice, 73
  definition of, 16, 20
  and EGD, 41
  "failed," 63

F

Famotidine, 58
Fatigue, and promotility drugs, 56
Fatty foods, as aggravating factor, 15, 53, 89, 104, 107
FDA (Food and Drug Administration)
  and Gaviscon, 56
  and new surgical procedures, 61, 62
  and PillCam ESO, 42
  and PPIs, xxviii
Fennel, as alternative treatment, 71
Fennel tea, as alternative treatment, 73
Fenugreek seeds
  as acid absorbers, 71
  as alternative treatment, 71
Feverfew, allergy to, and chamomile, 70–71
Fish (sole), spinach-stuffed, recipe for, 116–117

Flank steak, grill marinated, recipe for, 113–114
Flax, as alternative treatment, 71
Food(s)
    canned, in GERD-friendly diet, 106
    choice of, and GERD therapy, 53
    fatty, as aggravating factor, 15, 53, 89, 107
    fried, as aggravating factor, 107
    impaction of. *See* Impaction
    recipes for GERD sufferers, 107–122
    restaurants, and GERD-friendly dining, 107–108
    route of, through digestive tract, 19–21, 20f
    spicy, as aggravating factor, 15, 53, 89, 107
Food pipe. *See* Esophagus
Fosamax, as aggravating factor, 16
Fried foods, as aggravating factor, 107
Fruit, in GERD-friendly diet, 105–106, 106
"Full wrap" procedure, 63–64, 65f
Fundus, 63

G
Gall-bladder problems, in case study, 6–7
Gallstones, and avoidance of turmeric, 73
Garlic
    as alternative treatment, 72
    shallot as substitute for in recipes, 121
Gas
    and carminative medications, 71
    "gas bloat syndrome" after surgery, 65
    and linden flower tea, 75
    and TLESRs, 22
Gastric acid pump. *See* Proton pump
Gastrin receptor, 57
Gastrin receptor pathway, 20
Gastritis, alternative treatments for, 72
Gastroenterologists, pediatric, 79
Gastrointestinal tract. *See* Digestive system
Gastroscope, 41, 41f
Gatekeeper (surgical procedure), 62, 84
    definition of, 97
Gaviscon, 55
Gender
    and GERD, 1
    and incidence of erosive esophagitis, 28
    and incidence of esophageal cancer, 34
General Nutrition Center (GNC), on carminative medicines, 71
GERD (gastroesophageal reflux disease), 14, 87. *See also* NERD (non-erosive esophagitis); Symptoms of GERD
    aggravating factors
        lifestyle, 7, 15

Index

medicines, 15–16
and asthma, 13, 88, 90
in children, 79
case studies of, 1–7
causes of, xxv–xxvi, 88
and children, 79
chronic nature of, xxvi, 52
complications of, 27–36, 88
diagnosis of, 39–48
and the elderly, 79–80
erosive, 14
    grading scale for (1-4 or A-D), 14, 28, 29f
and esophageal stricture, 33
frequency of, 14, 15f
vs. heartburn, 87
and Helicobacter pylori bacteria, 77–78, 92
vs. hiatal hernia, 88
iceberg metaphor, xxvii, xxviii$f$
and infants, 79
non-erosive. See NERD (non-erosive esophagitis)
in pregnancy, 78–79
severity of, vs. severity of symptoms, 16, 27, 36, 42
in the elderly, 80
spelled GORD in Europe, xxv
sphincter incompetence and, 25
stress and, in case study, 4
TLESRs and, 22
universality of, 80–81
untreated, and incidence of Barrett's esophagus, 30
Ginger (Zingiber officinale)
as alternative treatment, 70–71, 72, 75
American Botanical Council and, 70
anti-inflammatory properties of, 70
anti-nausea properties of, 70, 72
intestinal movement and, 70
Globus (sensation of lump in throat), as symptom, 13
GORD, European spelling of GERD, xxv
Grading scale (1-4 or A-D), for esophageal erosion, 14, 28, 29f
Grains, in GERD-friendly diet, 104–105
Gravity
as defense against GERD, 22
and elderly patients, 80
and nocturnal reflux, 11, 24
Gravy, roasted onion and shallot, recipe for, 121–122
Gum, chewing, and reflux symptoms, 23
Gynecomastia (enlarged breasts), and Tagamet (cimetidine), 58

H

H_2 blockers, 55, 91
chemistry of, 57–58
definition of, 97
before meals, 53
and pregnancy, 78, 89
H_2RAs (H_2 receptor antagonists). See H_2 blockers

H_2 receptor, 57
H_2 receptor pathway, 20
Halitosis (bad breath), as symptom, 13–14
Headache
  and H_2RAs, 58
  and PPIs, 59
  and promotility drugs, 56
Heartburn
  alternative treatments for, 71, 73, 74
  and "bitter digestive stimulants," 71
  and boldo, 75
  and the elderly, 80
  mistaken for heart attack, 4, 9, 12–13
    in case study, 4
    first-person account of, 9
  in pregnancy, 78
    and hairy babies, 78
  prevalence of, xxv, 10
  and stomach bitters, 74
  as symptom of GERD, xxv–xxvi, 9–10, 87–88
Heart conditions, and licorice, 72–73
Heart-valves, artificial, and EGD, 42
Helicobacter pylori bacteria
  definition of, 97
  and GERD, 77–78, 92
  and ulcers, 77
Hemorrhage, and erosive esophagitis, 28
Herbal treatments. See Alternative and complementary treatments
Herbs. See also Alternative and complementary treatments
  dried, in GERD-friendly diet, 106
  fresh, in recipes, 109
Hernia, hiatal, 24–25, 24f
  and age, 80
  barium esophagram/upper gastrointestinal series test for, 46–47
  and Barrett's esophagus, 30–31
  in case studies, 3, 5
  causes of, 25
  confused with GERD, 24, 88
  confused with heartburn, 24
  as contributing or aggravating factor, 15, 23
  definition of, 98
  and endocinch procedure, 61
  first-person account of, 25
  and Nissen fundoplication, 63–64
  and Stretta procedure, 61
Hiccups, and GERD in infants, 79
High blood pressure, and licorice, 72–73
Histamine$_2$ blockers. See H_2 blockers
Histamine$_2$ receptor. See H_2 receptor
Histamine$_2$ receptor pathway. See H_2 receptor pathway
Hoarseness, as symptom, 14, 88
  in infants, 79

Index

Hydrochloric acid
   and GERD, 10
   secretion of, 20, 57
Hydrogen potassium adenosine triphosphate pump. *See* Proton pump

I

Impaction, food
   in case study, 2
   and esophageal stricture, 34
Impedance testing, 46, 48
Impotence, and Tagamet (cimetidine), 58
Inderal, as aggravating factor, 16
Indigestion. *See also* Digestion
   and artichoke, 75
   and boldo, 75
   and carminative medications, 71
   and centaurium, 74
   and green tea, 75
   and linden, 75
   and rosemary, 75
Infants, and GERD, 79
Infection
   bronchial, recurrent, as symptom, 13, 88
   of stomach lining, alternative treatments for, 71–72
Inflammation of stomach lining
   alternative treatments for, 71–72
   antacids and, 56
   and Helicobacter pylori bacteria, 92

Inflammatory disorders, licorice as alternative treatment for, 72
Insurance companies, and experimental procedures, 32, 61, 62
Interaction, between alternative and prescription medications, 70, 72
Intestinal irritation, and carminative medications, 71
Intestinal movement, and ginger, 70
Intestines, 19, 20*f*
   small, and PillCam ESO, 44
Irritability, nux vomica for, 74
Irritation, esophageal, and chamomile, 70

J

Johnson DeMeester Score, 45
Juices
   apple, in herbal teas, 71
   carrot, in herbal teas, 71
   citrus, as aggravating factor, 15, 53
   tomato, as aggravating factor, 15

K

Ketchup, in GERD-friendly diet, 106
Kidney problems
   and aluminum-related dementia, 60
   and licorice as alternative treatment, 72–73

L

Lamb loins, marinated, recipe for, 112–113
Lansoprazole, 58–59
Laryngitis, chronic, as symptom, 14
Lavender, as alternative treatment, 75
Lemon balm, as alternative treatment, 75
Lentils, in GERD-friendly diet, 105
LES (lower esophageal sphincter), 21–22, 21f, 24f
    definition of, 98
    hypotensive, 22–23
    malfunction of, and GERD, 22, 88
    pressure of, 21
        increased by promotility drugs, 56
    relaxation of, in the elderly, 80
    surgical procedures and, 61–62
    tightening of, by stomach bitters, 74
Lethargy, and promotility drugs, 56
Levodopa, as aggravating factor, 16
Licorice root (Glycyrrhiza glabra)
    as alternative treatment, 71–73
    dangers of high doses of, 72
Lifestyle, and GERD therapy, 7, 52–54
Linden and linden flower tea, as alternative treatment, 75
Liver
    and drug interactions, 60
    problems with, and licorice, 72–73
Lying down. *See* Position, body

M

Maalox, 2
Magee, Elaine, 89
Magnesium, in antacids, 55
Magnesium-based calcium carbonate, in antacids, 55
Maintenance therapy, 52
Malic acid, and stomach acid, 71
Malnourishment, and decreased resistance of esophageal mucosa, 24
Marshmallow, as alternative treatment, 71
Marshmallow root tea, as alternative treatment, 73
Medications
    as aggravating factor, 15–16, 54, 89
        anti-cholinergic, 16
        birth-control, 16
        bone-density, 16
    alternative. *See* Alternative and complementary treatments
    carminative, 71
    and elderly patients, 80
    first-person account of, 54
    maintenance *vs.* "on-demand," 52, 91

Index

over-the-counter, 25, 39, 43, 83
   in case studies, 2, 3–4
  and pregnancy, 78–79
   classification for (A, B, C, D, X), 78–79
  prescription, 25, 84
   in case studies, 4, 6
  spending on, xxvi, 51
Medicine
  Ayurvedic, and turmeric, 73
  botanical, practitioners of, 72
  Chinese, and turmeric, 73
Metastasis, and esophageal cancer, 35–36
Metoclopramide, 56
Michalski, Sue, case study of, 3–4, 3f
Motility
  esophageal
   decreased during sleep, 24
   testing of, 46, 47–48
  gut, and stomach bitters, 74
Motion sickness, and ginger, 72
Motrin, as aggravating factor, 16
Mucilage
  and heartburn, 74
  in slippery elm, 74
Mucosa, esophageal, decreased resistance of, 24
Muffins, corn, recipe for, 108–109
Multiple sclerosis, and delayed esophageal clearance, 23
Mushroom stuffing, wild, recipe for, 119–121
Mustard, in GERD-friendly diet, 106

N

Naprosyn, as aggravating factor, 16
Narcotics, as aggravating factor, 16
Narrowing of the esophagus. *See* Esophageal stricture
National Health Interview Survey, on alternative and complementary medicine, 69
National Heartburn Alliance, 104, 105, 107–108
  website, 125
Nausea
  ginger for, 72
  and H_2RAs, 58
  and linden, 75
  nux vomica for, 72
  and PPIs, 59
NDO plicator (surgical procedure), 61–62, 84
NERD (non-erosive esophagitis), 14, 28. *See also* GERD (gastroesophageal reflux disease)
  first-person account of, 48
  frequency of, 14, 15f
  not always mild, 14
  testing for, 44
Nexium, xxviii, 58–59
Nissen, Rudolph, 84
Nissen fundoplication (surgery), 63–64, 91
  definition of, 98
  "full wrap," 63, 65f
  history of, 84

"partial wrap" (toupet) procedure, 63–64, 66f, 99
   pros and cons of, 62–63
   risks and side effects of, 64–65
   tests to prepare for, 63
Nitrates, and hypotensive LES, 22–23
Nizatidine, 58
Noise and light, sensitivity to, nux vomica for, 74
Noninvasive methods, and screening for Barrett's esophagus, 33
Norvasc, as aggravating factor, 16
NSAIDs (e.g. aspirin, Motrin, Naprosyn), as aggravating factor, 16
Nux vomica, as alternative treatment, 74

O

Obesity
   as aggravating factor, 15, 54, 89
      in case study, 3
   epidemic of, 3
   and increased intra-abdominal pressure, 24
   and licorice as alternative treatment, 72–73
Octasulphate, 60
Odonophagia (pain with swallowing)
   definition of, 98
   and esophageal stricture, 33–34
   and GERD diagnosis, 40
   as sign of complications, 11
   as symptom, 11, 88
Oesaphagus (European spelling). *See* Esophagus
Oils, in food
   as aggravating factor, 104, 107
   in GERD-friendly diet, 105
Omeprazole, 58–59
Onions
   raw, as aggravating factor, 15, 89
   roasted onion and shallot gravy, recipe for, 121–122
   Vidalia, easier on digestion, 115, 121
Oregano, as alternative treatment, 75
Overeating, and sour burps, 74

P

Pacemakers, and Bravo pH Monitoring System, 45
Pain
   abdominal, and PPIs, 59
   chest. *See* Chest pain
   epigastric (upper abdominal), as symptom, 11, 88
Pantaprozole, 59
Papaya and papaya seeds, as alternative treatment, 75
Papaya enzyme, chewable tablets of, 75
Papaya tea, as alternative treatment, 73
Parkinson's disease, medications for, as aggravating factor, 16

Index

Parks, Carlene, case study of, 6–7, 6f
"Partial wrap" (toupet) procedure, 63–64, 66f, 99
Pasta
   bow-tie, with peas and ham, recipe for, 109–111
   in GERD-friendly diet, 105
PDT (photodynamic therapy), 32, 35, 84
   definition of, 98–99
Peas, in GERD-friendly diet, 105
Pectin
   in Aloe vera juice, 73
   and GERD, 73
Pepcid, xxviii, 58
   and pregnancy, 78
Peppermint
   as aggravating factor, 15, 53, 89
   as alternative treatment, 71
   and hypotensive LES, 22–23
Peristalsis, 20, 20f
   and age, 80
   as defense against GERD, 22
   definition of, 98
   and gum chewing, 23
   inadequate or uncoordinated, 46–47
   and nocturnal reflux, 11–12
   and promotility drugs, 56
   and surgery, 63
pH monitoring. See Bravo pH Monitoring System
Photodynamic therapy. See PDT
Photosensitizing drugs, in PDT, 32
Phrenicoesophageal ligament, 22
   definition of, 99
PillCam ESO, xxix, 40, 42–44, 43f, 90, 91
   definition of, 99
   and EGD followup, 43
   and screening for Barrett's esophagus, 33
Pineapple, as alternative treatment, 75
Plavix, and EGD, 42
Plication (stitch), 61–62
Porfimer sodium, in PDT, 32
Position, body
   and age, 80
   in case studies, 3, 4
   and GERD therapy, 53–54
PPIs (proton pump inhibitors), xxviii, 51, 55, 58–60, 84, 91
   chemistry of, 57
   definition of, 98
   dosage of, 59
   interactions with Coumadin, Valium, Digoxin, and Biaxin, 60
   before meals, 53
   in pregnancy, 78–79
   side effects of, 59–60
Pregnancy
   as aggravating factor for GERD, 15, 89
   and avoidance of centaurium, 73
   and avoidance of dill, 73

heartburn and GERD in, 78–79
    first-person account of, 79
and increased intra-abdominal
    pressure, 24
medications and, 78–79
    classification for (A, B, C, D,
    X), 78–79
Prevacid, xxviii, 58–59
Prilosec, 51, 58–59
    and pregnancy, 79
Procardia, as aggravating factor,
    16
Promotility (prokinetic) drugs, 55,
    56–57, 91
    definition of, 99
    side effects of, 56
Propulsid, 56–57
Prosthesis, artificial, and EGD, 42
Protonix, xxviii, 59
Proton pump, 57, 57*f*
Provocative testing, 46, 48
Pylorus, 21

Q

Quality of life
    and GERD, xxvi, xxviii, 1, 83
    and nocturnal reflux, 12

R

Rabeprazole, 59
Race
    and GERD, 1
    and incidence of Barrett's
        esophagus, 30
    and incidence of erosive
        esophagitis, 28
    and incidence of esophageal
        cancer, 34
Ragweed allergy, and chamomile,
    70–71
Ranitidine, 58
Recipes, for GERD sufferers,
    107–122
Reflux, acid
    and bicarbonate in saliva, 11
    body's defenses against, 22
    in case studies, 1–4, 6–7
    and green tea, 75
    nocturnal
        vs. daytime, 11–12
        first-person account of, 12
        and quality of life, 1, 12
        as symptom, 11–12
    and stomach bitters, 74
Reglan, 56
Regurgitation
    first-person account of, 11
    as symptom, xxvi, 11, 88
Relapse rates, GERD *vs.* NERD, 52
Restaurants, and GERD-friendly
    dining, 107–108
Retching without vomiting, nux
    vomica for, 74
Rigidity, and promotility drugs,
    56
Rolaids, 3
Rosemary, as alternative treatment, 75

S

Sage, as alternative treatment, 75

Index

Salad, herbed orzo, with corn, recipe for, 111–112
Salad dressings, oil-based, as aggravating factor, 107
Salbutamol, as aggravating factor, 16
Saliva
    bicarbonate in, and nocturnal reflux, 11
    decreased production of, 23
    as defense against GERD, 22
Salivation
    decreased during sleep, 24
    and gum chewing, 23
    and nocturnal reflux, 11
Sauces, in GERD-friendly diet, 105
Scar tissue, and esophageal stricture, 33–34
Scleroderma, and delayed esophageal clearance, 23
Screening
    guidelines for, 33
    periodic, and dysplasia, 30
Sedatives, as aggravating factor, 16
Self-diagnosis, 39
Self-knowledge
    and personal diet, 103–104
    and restaurant menus, 107
    and symptoms of GERD, 17
Self-medication, 39
    in case study, 4
Sensitivity to noise and light, nux vomica for, 74
"Sewing" (surgery). *See* Endocinch procedure

Shallot, as substitute for garlic, 121
Side effects
    of alternative medications, 72
    of antacids, 55–56
Signs of GERD. *See* Symptoms of GERD
Skin diseases, licorice as alternative treatment for, 72
Sleep apnea, possibly related to GERD, 14
Sleep difficulties
    and GERD, xxvi
    in infants, 79
    and nocturnal reflux, 12
Sleeping on left side, 53
Slippery elm
    as alternative treatment, 71–72, 74
    mucilage in, 74
Smoking
    as aggravating factor, 15, 54, 89
    and decreased salivary production, 23
Soda (caffeinated), as aggravating factor, 15, 53, 89, 107
Sodium bicarbonate, in antacids, 55
Soft drinks (caffeinated), as aggravating factor, 15, 53, 89, 107
Sole, spinach-stuffed, recipe for, 116–117
Sore throat
    chronic, as symptom, 14

licorice as alternative treatment for, 72
Sour burps. *See also* Belching
  causes of, 74
  nux vomica for, 74
Sphincter
  lower esophageal. *See* LES (lower esophageal sphincter)
  upper esophageal, 20
Spices and herbs, in GERD-friendly diet, 106
Spicy foods, as aggravating factor, 15, 89, 107
Spinach-stuffed sole, recipe for, 116–117
St. John's wort, as alternative treatment, 72
Steak, grill marinated flank, recipe for, 113–114
Stomach, 19, 21*f*, 24*f*
  and EGD, 41
  and PillCam ESO, 44
Stress, and GERD, in case study, 4
Stretta procedure (surgical), 61, 84, 91
  definition of, 99
Stricture, esophageal. *See* Esophageal stricture
"Stuffing" (surgical procedure). *See* Enteryx, injection with
Stuffing, wild mushroom, recipe for, 119–121
Submucosal resection. *See* Endoscopic mucosal resection
Sucralfate, 60
Surgery
  and Barrett's esophagus, 65–66
  in case studies, 4, 5
  endoscopic procedures, 61–62
  for esophageal cancer, 35, 65–66
  and esophageal motility testing, 47–48
  and esophageal stricture, 65–66
  laparoscopic, 62, 91
    definition of, 98
  Nissen fundoplication. *See* Nissen fundoplication
Swallowing
  difficulty with. *See* Dysphagia
  pain with. *See* Odonophagia
Sweating, as symptom, in case study, 5
Sweet potatoes and summer vegetables, roasted, recipe for, 115–116
Symptoms of GERD, 9–15, 88
  atypical, 10
  breakthrough, 55
  chronic, and testing, 39, 40
  inconsistency of, 16–17
  self-knowledge and, 17
  severity of, *vs.* severity of disease, 16, 27, 36, 42
  typical, 10
  uncommon, 10

T

Tachyphylaxis, 58
Tagamet, xxviii, 58
  and gynecomastia (enlarged breasts), 58
  and impotence, 58

Index

and pregnancy, 78
Tardive dyskinesia, and promotility drugs, 56
Tartaric acid, and stomach acid, 71
Tea
   green, as alternative treatment, 75
   herbal, as alternative treatment, 73
   as sometimes aggravating factor, 15, 53, 89, 107
Tell Me What to Eat If I Have Acid Reflux (Magee), 89, 104
Tenormin, as aggravating factor, 16
Terbutaline, as aggravating factor, 16
Testing
   for GERD, 39–48
   impedance, 46, 48
   provocative, 46, 48
Theophylline
   as aggravating factor, 16
   and hypotensive LES, 22–23
Therapy, photodynamic. *See* PDT
Thistle, blessed, as alternative treatment, 71
Thyme, as alternative treatment, 75
TLESR (transient lower esophageal sphincter relaxation)
   definition of, 22, 99–100
   gas and, 22
   GERD and, 22
Tofranil, as aggravating factor, 16
Tomato products, as aggravating factor, 15, 89, 107, 109
Tooth decay, 14*f*
   as symptom, 13, 88
Toupet ("partial wrap") procedure, 63–64, 66*f*, 99
Treatment
   goals of, 52
   maintenance *vs.* "on-demand," 52, 91
Tremors, and promotility drugs, 56
Tricyclic antidepressants, as aggravating factor, 16
Trocar (surgical tool), 65
Tuberculosis, licorice as alternative treatment for, 72
Tums, 2, 79
Turmeric (Curcuma longa)
   as alternative treatment, 73
   and ulcers, 73

U

Ulcers
   and dosage of turmeric, 73
   esophageal, 28
      first-person account of, 28
   and esophageal stricture, 33
   and Helicobacter pylori bacteria, 92
   and PillCam ESO, 44

V

Vagus nerve, and acid secretion, 20

Valium
    as aggravating factor, 16
    interactions with PPIs, 60
Vegetables, summer, roasted with sweet potatoes, recipe for, 115–116
Ventolin, as aggravating factor, 16
Vinegar, in GERD-friendly diet, 105–106
Volmax, as aggravating factor, 16
Vomiting
    and esophageal cancer, 35
    and GERD diagnosis, 40
        in infants and children, 79
        during pregnancy, 79

W
Waterbrash (excess salivation), as symptom, 11, 88
Websites, recommended, 125–127

Weight gain, as aggravating factor, 15
Weight loss
    and esophageal cancer, 35
    and GERD diagnosis, 40
        in children, 79
Wormwood, as alternative treatment, 71
Wurm, Charles, case study of, 1–3, 2*f*

Y
Yam, wild, as alternative treatment, 72

Z
Zantac, xxviii, 58
    and pregnancy, 78
Zegerid, xxviii, 59
Zelnorm, 56–57

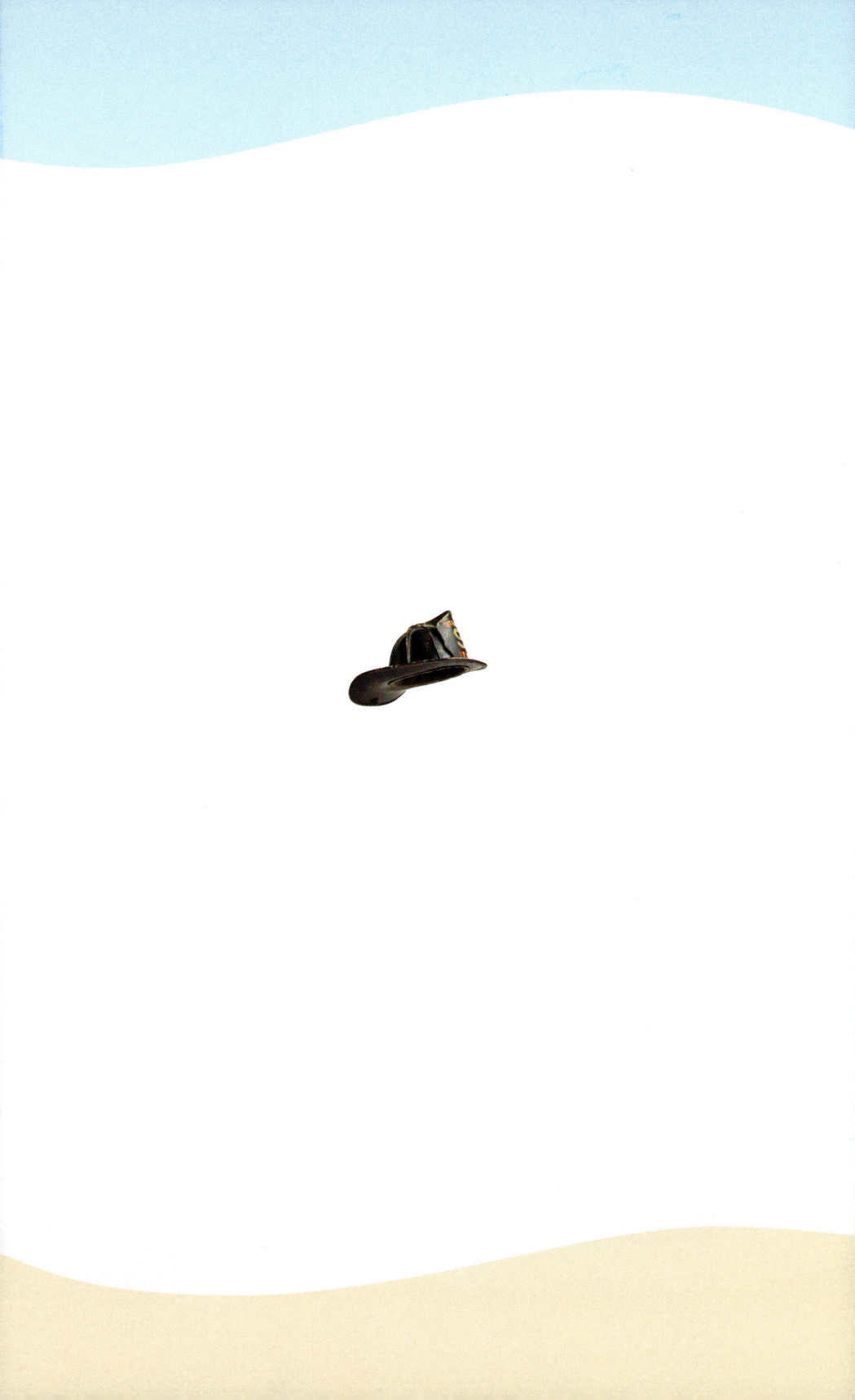

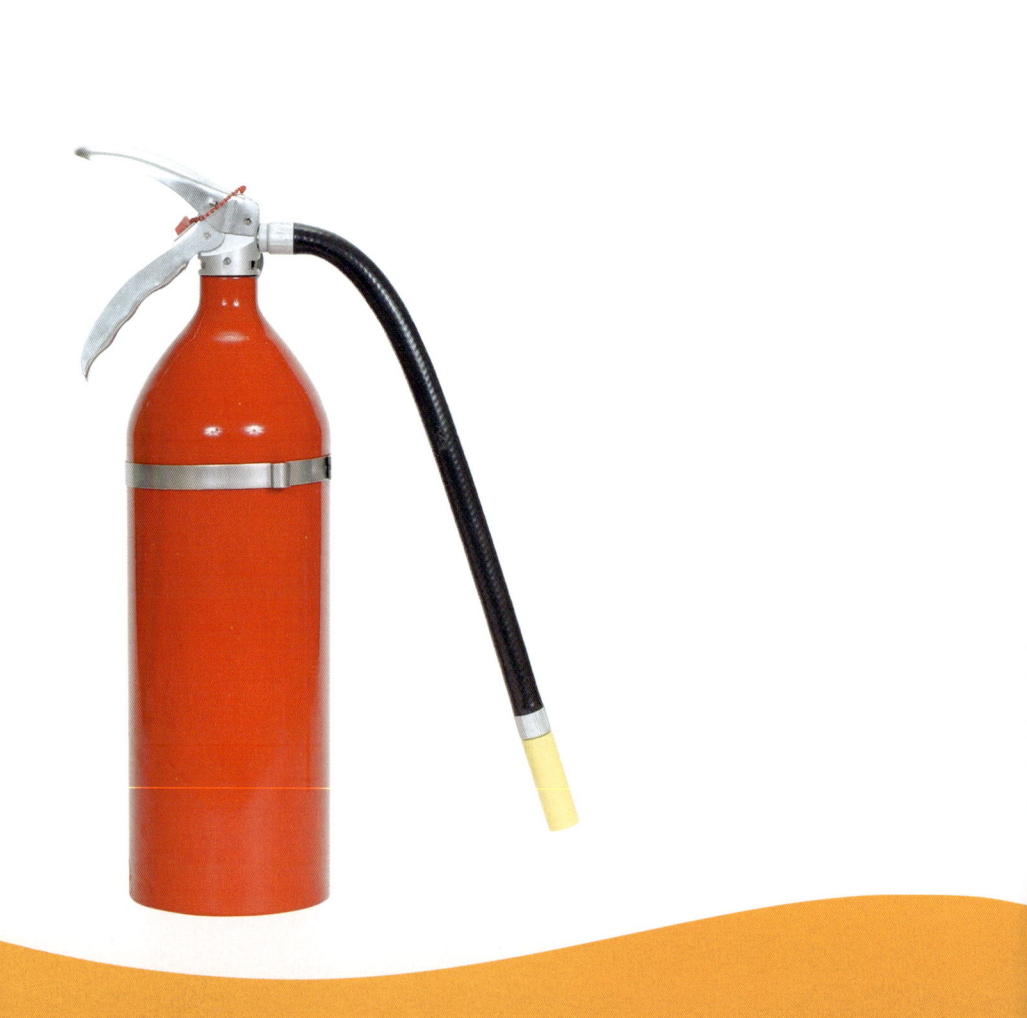

Special Thanks

Bergein Overholt, M.D.
Joel Richter, M.D.
Morgan Chilson
Shelby Herbers
Nancy Sousa, Given Imaging
Rao Donepudi, M.D.
Vijay Mhatre, M.D.
Jerry Feagan, M.D.
Sally Taylor
Sandy Shuster, Medtronic
Mark Traffas, Medtronic
Linda Miller, National Heartburn Alliance
Nason Lui, M.D.
Tahira Saifuddin, M.D.

Spurn the Burn

Parminder Chawla, M.D.
Bernita Berntsen, M.D., Midwest Heartburn Clinic
Carlyle Dunshee, M.D., Midwest heartburn Clinic
Padma Raju, M.D.
Jayalakshmi Pampati, M.D.
Kalpana Miryala, M.D.
Malini Pampati, M.D.
Elaine Magee, The Recipe Doctor
Ginger Disney, Given Imaging
Rama Lakshmi Donepudi
Mike Ruffalo, Salix Pharmaceuticals
Cindy Feagan, ARNP
Stephanie Jernigan, ARNP
Charlie Wurm, P.A.-C.
Laura Welborn, ARNP
Jill Scheuler, P.A.-C.
James Balch, P.A.-C.
Holly Balch
Michelle Meier
Mary Baumgartner
Cori Wegner
Sue Michalski
Jim Kline
Carlene Parks
Rebecca Dennison
Patti Best
Chony Ayala
Charlene Urton
Vicki Henderson
Melinda Gooch

Special Thanks

Janet McKee
Staci Valdivia
Jenny Panone
Barbara Khalil
Cara Bagby
Karthik Challa
Supriya Challa
Ashwin Pampati
Rudra Pampati
Jenny Walker
Vicki Hufford
Heidi Hughes
Diana Harty
Amy Sloop
Jane Ziegler
Pam Partridge
Kay Brumbaugh
Theresa Hicks
Colleen Bane
Connie Brackey
Amy Ewing
Tracy Halvenstein
Evelyn Huggins
Laura Lewis
Stacy McCrory
Sherry Selk
Susan Smith
Robin Murray
The Pneuma Books Team — Brian, Mike, Nina, Heather, Jane, and Sarah

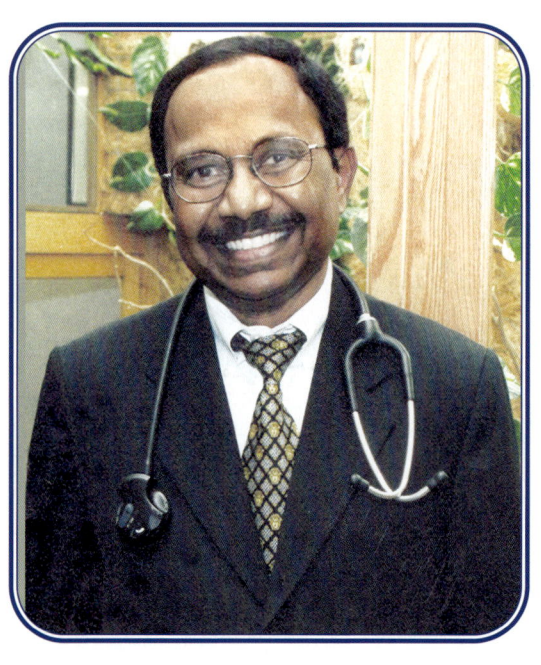

About the Author

Dr. Shekhar Challa has been on the forefront of gastroenterology and hepatology for eighteen years. In private practice in Topeka since 1987, Dr. Challa is the Medical Director for the Midwest Heartburn Clinic, President of Kansas Medical Clinic, and CEO of Osteoporosis Services.

He is a featured speaker for The Chronic Liver Disease Foundation and is also on numerous boards, including the West Central Osteoporosis Board of Proctor and Gamble, an Alliance for Better Bone Health, US Bank, and My Medical Records.com, Inc.

Dr. Challa is also the author of *Winning the Hepatitis C Battle,* which was a Ben Franklin finalist and a 2003 Reader's Preference Editor's Choice Award finalist.

My Healing Helpers

Winning the Hepatitis C Battle

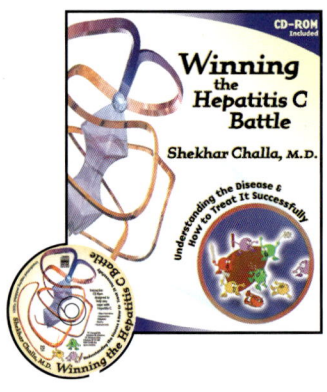

Awards

- Reader's Preference Editor's Choice Award Finalist, 2003
- Benjamin Franklin Finalist, 2004

What Others Are Saying...

"This should be required for patients and their families. It's practical and guides the reader in taking control of their lives."
— Barbara Veres, *Hepatitis* Magazine

"The book and CD cover every topic related to Hepatitis C. I highly recommend it."
— Alan Franciscus, Exec. Dir., *Hepatitis C Support Project* and Editor-in Chief, HCV Advocate

"This book is written in a direct and easily understandable manner. The lay public interested in Hepatitis C will benefit from a close reading of this book."
— Dr. Michael Sorrell, Robert L. Grissom Professor of Medicine, University of Nebraska

To order, visit www.hepcbattle.com or call 866-746-1448 toll-free.

◉📕💿💻 **My Healing Helpers**

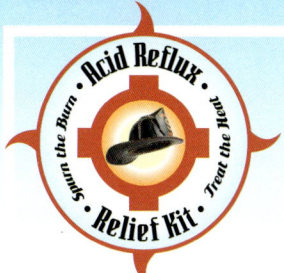

Acid Reflux Relief Kit

www.acidrefluxreliefkit.com

Each Kit Contains

- An acid reflux relief pillow
- *Spurn the Burn, Treat the Heat: Everything You Need to Know to Beat Acid Reflux Disease* by Shekhar Challa, M.D.
- *Tell Me What to Eat If I Have Acid Reflux* and *Fry Light, Fry Right* by Elaine Magee, The Recipe Doctor
- The Heartburn-Friendly Kitchen — A DVD on acid reflux and GERD. With an update by Dr. Shekhar Challa and dietary tips and recipes by Elaine Magee, The Recipe Doctor
- Chat with Challa audio CD
- Access to Spurn the Burn teleconferences — during these scheduled teleconferences, patients can listen to experts discuss GERD and offer solutions for living with this condition
- A free subscription to the e-mail newsletter, Acid Reflux Insider
- Membership in the Reflux Recipe of the Month Club — a new recipe will be e-mailed to you each month
- Brochures and educational information from various resources — including coupons and/or medication samples

Check the website for availability. Contents of the kit subject to change without notice.

◉❚📖🖳 **My Healing Helpers**

Ordering Information

For more information on books from My Healing Helpers call 866-746-1448 toll-free or visit:

www.spurntheburn.com

My Healing Helper books, kits, DVDs, and other resources are available online or at your favorite bookstore.

Quantity discounts are available to qualifying institutions.

Dr. Challa's books are available to the booktrade and other groups through all major wholesalers.

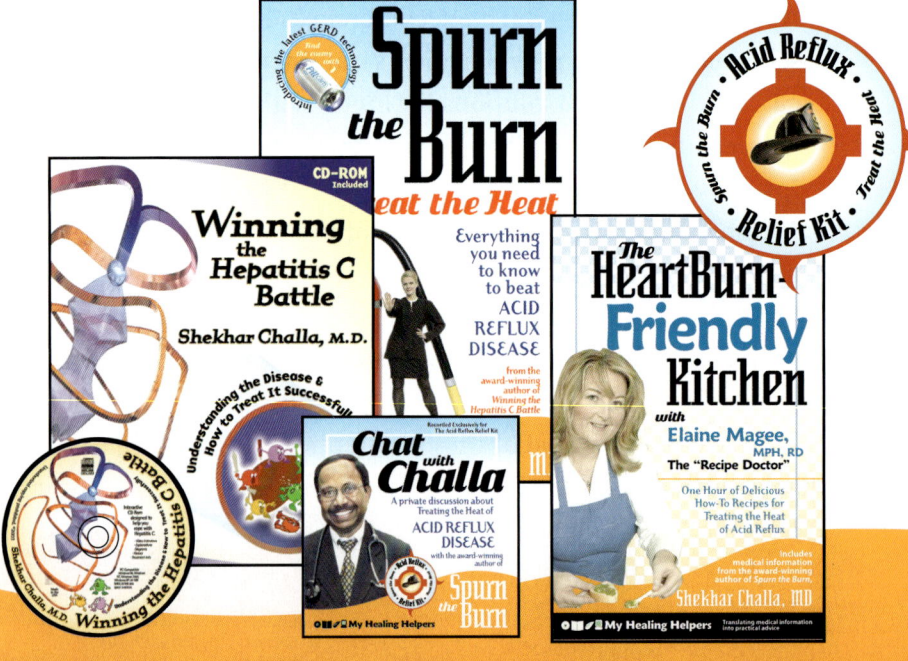

My Healing Helpers

spurntheburn.com

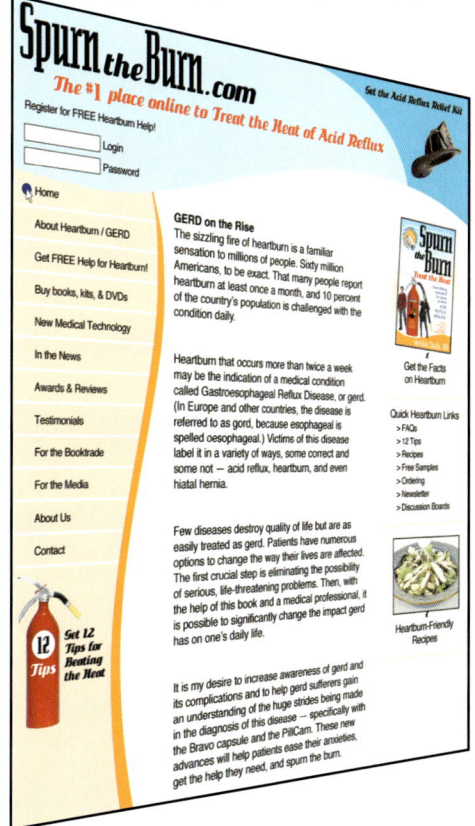

Register here for weekly drawings of the Acid Reflux Relief Kit and a free subscription to the Acid Reflux Insider, a monthly e-mail newsletter.

If you don't have web access but would still like to be entered into our weekly drawing for an Acid Reflux Relief Kit, print your full name and address on a 3 x 5 card and mail it to: Kansas Medical Publishing, 2200 SW 6th Ave., Suite 104, Topeka, KS 66606 or call us at 866-746-1448.

We will not share personal information, all information is strictly confidential.

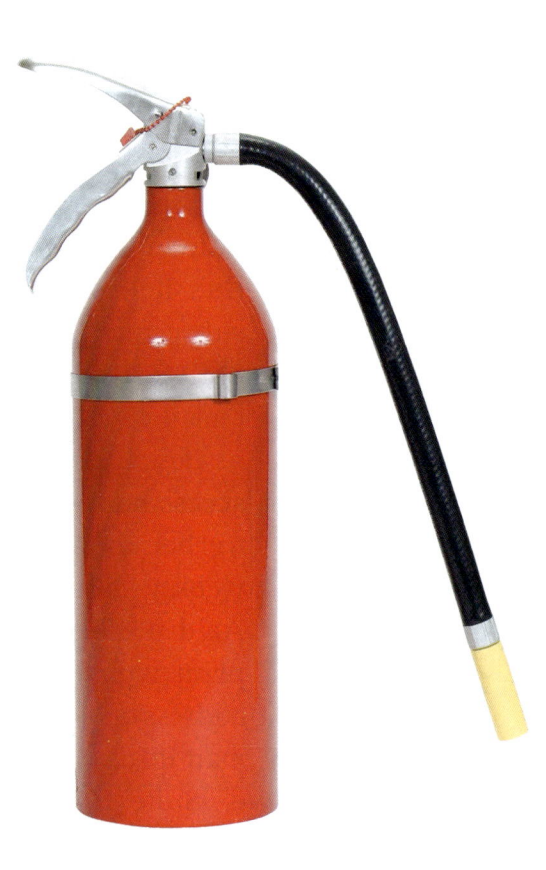